# CNA

# *Nursing Assistant Certification Exam*

# *Prep Textbook*

### Unlock Your Potential and Conquer the CNA Exam with Ease and Empowered Strategies

2024-25
EDITION

MasterProLearning101 Publications - Nathan Yarbridge

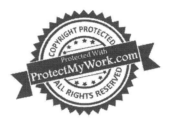

# UNLOCK ESSENTIAL EXTRA STUDY TOOLS!

Before diving into the chapters,
**SCAN THE QR CODE at the end of this book**
to access a suite of valuable resources — including:

> ➢ **AUDIO CLIPS**
>
> ➢ **FLASHCARDS**
>
> ➢ **STUDY GUIDES**
>
> ➢ **EXTRA TESTS**

These materials are designed to significantly enhance your learning experience. **Download them immediately** to ensure you don't miss out on these **crucial aids for your CNA exam preparation.**

## *DON'T MISS OUT ON YOUR STUDY BOOSTERS!*

Scan the QR code and join the facebook page CNA Nursing Assistant Exam Prep Certification

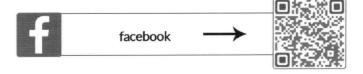

# Table of contents

UNLOCK ESSENTIAL EXTRA STUDY TOOLS! ........................................................................................................3

**Introduction** ........................................................................................................................................... 11

**Chapter 1: Foundations of Care** ........................................................................................................... 13

Understanding the Role of the Nurse Aide ........................................................................................... 13

Legal Considerations for Nurse Aides ................................................................................................... 14

    HIPAA Privacy Rules ............................................................................................................................ 14

    Affordable Care Act and Changes to Reimbursement Models ........................................................... 14

    CMS Regulations for Nursing Homes ................................................................................................. 14

    OSHA Standards for Workplace Safety .............................................................................................. 14

    Emerging Policies as Value-Based Care Models ................................................................................ 15

    Right to Informed Consent and Shared Decision-Making .................................................................. 15

    Right to Privacy, Dignity, and Respect ............................................................................................... 15

    Right to Freedom from Abuse, Neglect or Mistreatment ................................................................... 15

    Right to Access Records and Transparent Billing .............................................................................. 15

    Accurately Recording Vital Signs, Intake/Outputs, ADLs .................................................................. 16

    Completing Forms, Charts, and Hourly Rounding Records ............................................................... 16

    Following Proper Chain of Command for Concerns ........................................................................... 16

    Understanding Do-Not-Resuscitate Orders ....................................................................................... 16

Ethical Principles in Healthcare .............................................................................................................. 16

    Autonomy and Respect for Persons ................................................................................................... 17

    Beneficence and Promoting Good ...................................................................................................... 17

    Nonmaleficence and Avoiding Harm .................................................................................................. 17

    Equal Treatment for All Patients ......................................................................................................... 17

    Fair Resource Allocation Without Discrimination ............................................................................... 18

    Advocating for vulnerable or marginalized groups ............................................................................. 18

    Reporting Illegal or Unethical Conduct .............................................................................................. 18

    Identifying and Analyzing Ethical Issues ............................................................................................ 18

    Weighing Alternative Solutions and Consequences .......................................................................... 18

    Collaborating with Team to Address Conflicts .................................................................................... 18

Documenting Objective Facts and Any Actions Taken ............................................................ 18

Reporting Unresolved Concerns Properly ........................................................................... 19

Effective Communication in Healthcare ................................................................................. 19

Active Listening and Focused Attention ............................................................................. 19

Clear Articulation Using Plain Language ........................................................................... 19

Open-Ended Questioning and Empathy ............................................................................. 19

Therapeutic Touch When Appropriate ............................................................................... 20

Cultural Differences in Spatial Boundaries ....................................................................... 20

Effective Clinical Documentation ...................................................................................... 20

Organizing Notes Chronologically and Objectively ............................................................ 20

Timely Completion of Forms, Reports and Records ........................................................... 20

Necessary Conciseness Balanced with Detail ................................................................... 20

**Chapter 2: Safety Procedures** ............................................................................................. **21**

Importance of Infection Control ............................................................................................. 21

Proper Hand Hygiene Techniques ..................................................................................... 21

Use of Personal Protective Equipment .............................................................................. 21

Disinfection of Equipment ................................................................................................. 22

Safe Injection Practices ..................................................................................................... 22

Isolation Precautions ......................................................................................................... 22

Emergency Protocols and First Aid ....................................................................................... 22

Responding To Changes in Condition ................................................................................ 22

Scene Safety ...................................................................................................................... 23

Choking/Obstructed Airway ............................................................................................... 23

Cardiopulmonary Resuscitation (CPR) .............................................................................. 23

Bleeding Emergencies ....................................................................................................... 23

Identifying and Reporting Abuse ........................................................................................... 24

Signs of Abuse ................................................................................................................... 24

Reporting Procedures ........................................................................................................ 24

Maintaining Confidentiality ................................................................................................ 24

Preventing Retaliation ........................................................................................................ 25

**Chapter 3: Promoting Health and Wellness** ......................................................................... **27**

Basics of Human Anatomy and Physiology ................................................................. 27

    Integumentary System .............................................................................................. 27

    Musculoskeletal System ........................................................................................... 27

    Circulatory System .................................................................................................... 28

    Respiratory System ................................................................................................... 28

    Nervous System ........................................................................................................ 28

    Endocrine System ..................................................................................................... 29

    Urinary System .......................................................................................................... 29

    Digestive System ....................................................................................................... 30

    Reproductive System ................................................................................................. 30

Understanding Residents' Rights ............................................................................... 30

    Privacy and Confidentiality ....................................................................................... 31

    Respect and Freedom from Abuse .......................................................................... 31

    Information Sharing and Consent ............................................................................. 31

    Complaints and Grievances ...................................................................................... 31

    Refusal of Treatment ................................................................................................ 32

    End-of-Life Choices .................................................................................................. 32

Nutrition, Hydration, and Feeding Techniques .......................................................... 32

    Components Of Nutrition Care Plans ........................................................................ 32

    The Normal Swallow Process ................................................................................... 33

    Dysphagia Signs and Symptoms ............................................................................. 33

    Altered Diets and Appropriate Food Textures .......................................................... 33

    Adaptive Devices for Feeding Assistance ................................................................ 34

    Proper Feeding Techniques ...................................................................................... 34

    Importance of Rapport in Care Tasks ...................................................................... 34

    Snack and Meal Service Protocols .......................................................................... 34

    Nourishments and Between Meal Offerings ............................................................. 35

    Common Dietary Restrictions ................................................................................... 35

**Chapter 4: Essential Nursing Skills** ......................................................................... 37

Recording Vital Signs: Procedures and Best Practices ............................................. 37

    Measuring Oral Temperature .................................................................................... 37

Measuring Radial Pulse .................................................................................................... 38

Measuring Respiratory Rate ........................................................................................... 38

Measuring Blood Pressure .............................................................................................. 39

Patterns and Documentation .......................................................................................... 39

Infection Control ............................................................................................................. 39

Principles of Body Mechanics ............................................................................................... 40

Centering And Balance .................................................................................................... 40

Back Care Principles ........................................................................................................ 40

Patient Transfers and Ambulation ................................................................................. 40

Bed Mobility and Positioning ......................................................................................... 41

Body Mechanics in Daily Tasks ...................................................................................... 41

Safe Lifting Fundamentals .............................................................................................. 41

Care of the Environment and Patient Belongings ............................................................... 41

Bed Making ...................................................................................................................... 41

Patient Room Cleaning .................................................................................................... 42

Daily and Terminal Cleaning ........................................................................................... 42

Isolation Room Cleaning ................................................................................................. 42

Responsible Item Storage ............................................................................................... 43

Handling Personal Belongings ........................................................................................ 43

**Chapter 5: Personal Care Proficiencies** ........................................................................... 45

Assisting with Activities of Daily Living (ADLs) ............................................................. 45

Bathing Patients .............................................................................................................. 45

Oral Hygiene and Denture Care ..................................................................................... 45

Hair Care and Grooming ................................................................................................. 45

Toileting and Incontinence Care .................................................................................... 46

Bed Mobility and Transfers ............................................................................................ 46

Range of Motion and Positioning ................................................................................... 46

Grooming and Hygiene Protocols ........................................................................................ 46

Nail Care ........................................................................................................................... 46

Shaving Patients .............................................................................................................. 47

Skin Care .......................................................................................................................... 47

Proper Hand Hygiene ......................................................................................................... 47

Dressing, Undressing, and Comfort Measures ........................................................................ 47

Considerations for Dressing/Undressing ............................................................................. 48

Shirts and Pants ............................................................................................................... 48

Socks and Shoes .............................................................................................................. 48

Robes, Gowns, and Briefs ................................................................................................ 48

Comfort Devices and Positions .......................................................................................... 49

Lifts And Transfers ........................................................................................................... 49

**Chapter 6: Mental and Social Care Needs** ............................................................................. 51

Addressing Psychological Changes in Aging ........................................................................... 51

Understanding the Aging Process ...................................................................................... 51

Emotional Needs of Elderly Patients .................................................................................. 51

Dealing with Grief and Loss .............................................................................................. 51

Empathy and Communication ............................................................................................ 52

Promoting Mental Well-Being ........................................................................................... 52

Emotional Intelligence in Care .......................................................................................... 52

The Impact of Stress on Aging Patients ............................................................................. 52

Dignity and Respect ......................................................................................................... 52

Strategies for Managing Challenging Behaviors ...................................................................... 52

Approaches to Cognitive Impairments and Dementia Care ....................................................... 53

Dementia: A Comprehensive Overview ............................................................................... 53

Person-Centered Care ......................................................................................................... 54

Creating A Supportive Environment .................................................................................... 54

Communication Strategies ................................................................................................ 54

**Chapter 7: Basic Restorative Services** ................................................................................... 55

Implementing Range of Motion Exercises .............................................................................. 55

Understanding Range of Motion Exercises .......................................................................... 55

CNA's Role in Implementing ROM Exercises ....................................................................... 55

Ambulation and Use of Assistive Devices .............................................................................. 56

Gait Training Protocols ..................................................................................................... 56

Transfer Techniques ................................................................................................................ 57

Ambulation Aids ..................................................................................................................... 57

Monitoring Vital Signs ............................................................................................................ 58

Documenting Progress ........................................................................................................... 58

Offering Encouragement ........................................................................................................ 58

Working as a Team.................................................................................................................. 59

Additional Training Opportunities .......................................................................................... 59

Complication Prevention: Ulcers, Contractures, and More ......................................................... 59

Pressure Ulcer Prevention...................................................................................................... 59

Nutritional Monitoring ........................................................................................................... 60

Environmental Modification.................................................................................................... 60

Prompt Wound Treatment ...................................................................................................... 60

Bowel/Bladder Regularity....................................................................................................... 61

Shared Vigilance ..................................................................................................................... 61

Patient Education .................................................................................................................... 61

**Chapter 8: Skills Evaluation Masterclass** ................................................................................ **63**

Preparing for the Practical Test................................................................................................... 63

Gaining Confidence Through Practice ..................................................................................... 63

Understanding The Evaluation Process ................................................................................... 63

Preparing Your Mindset .......................................................................................................... 64

Organizing Your Resources ..................................................................................................... 64

Test-Day Etiquette and Conduct ............................................................................................. 65

Demonstrating Core Skills: Step-by-Step Breakdown ................................................................. 66

Hand Hygiene ......................................................................................................................... 66

Assisting with Activities of Daily Living (ADLs)........................................................................ 67

Vital Signs Measurement ........................................................................................................ 67

Assisting with Mobility ........................................................................................................... 68

Infection Control ..................................................................................................................... 69

Expert Tips and Common Pitfalls ................................................................................................ 70

**Chapter 9: Exam Strategy and Test-Taking Skills**.................................................................... **71**

Navigating Multiple Choice Questions: Tips and Tricks ..................................................................... 71

Time Management Techniques ................................................................................................... 71

Overcoming Test Anxiety ........................................................................................................ 72

**Chapter 10: Comprehensive Practice Questions and Scenarios** ..................................................... 73

Exam Test Training.................................................................................................................. 73

EXAM 1 ............................................................................................................................. 74

EXAM 2 ............................................................................................................................. 78

EXAM 3 ............................................................................................................................. 82

EXAM 4 ............................................................................................................................. 86

EXAM 1 - CORRECT ANSWERS............................................................................................. 91

EXAM 2 - CORRECT ANSWERS............................................................................................. 94

EXAM 3 - CORRECT ANSWERS............................................................................................. 97

EXAM 4 - CORRECT ANSWERS........................................................................................... 100

Practical Skill Scenarios for Hands-On Preparation ...................................................................... 103

Sample Skills Scenario #1 ...................................................................................................... 103

Sample Skills Scenario #2 ...................................................................................................... 103

Sample Skills Scenario #3 ...................................................................................................... 104

**Conclusion** ........................................................................................................................ 105

**EXTRA CONTENT DOWNLOAD**............................................................................................. 107

# Introduction

This comprehensive textbook is your indispensable companion on the path to becoming a Certified Nursing Assistant (CNA), arming you with the knowledge and skills essential for success in the dynamic field of healthcare.

Begin your exploration with the foundational elements of care, where legal considerations, ethical principles, and effective communication strategies set the stage for ethical and lawful healthcare practices. Dive into safety procedures, emphasizing infection control, proper hand hygiene, and emergency protocols, ensuring your readiness to respond to changes in patient conditions and identify/report abuse.

You will then shift towards promoting health and wellness, delving into human anatomy and physiology, residents' rights, and the intricate details of nutrition, hydration, and feeding techniques. Develop essential nursing skills, honing proficiency in vital sign recording, infection control, body mechanics, and environmental care.

Navigate the realm of personal care, mastering activities of daily living, commonly known as ADLs, such as, oral hygiene, bathing, grooming, and toileting. Explore the nuances of mental and social care needs, addressing psychological changes of aging, challenging behaviors, and cognitive impairments.

Advance to basic restorative services, implementing a range of motion exercises, promoting independence through ambulation, and preventing complications like pressure ulcers. The textbook culminates in a skills evaluation masterclass, guiding you through the practical test with step-by-step breakdowns, expert tips, and common pitfalls to avoid.

Sharpen your exam strategy and test-taking skills with insights on navigating multiple-choice questions, managing time effectively, and overcoming test anxiety. Finally, immerse yourself in a comprehensive set of practice questions and hands-on scenarios, mirroring the exam format to reinforce your knowledge and provide a realistic test-taking experience.

This textbook is not just a guide to passing certification exams—it's a gateway to excellence in your role as a healthcare professional. Each section is crafted to bridge the gap between theory and application, equipping you with the confidence and competence needed to excel in the diverse and rewarding field of healthcare. Embrace this educational journey, knowing that you are supported by a resource designed to empower you in your pursuit of excellence. Let the learning unfold.

Disclaimer: Although this book aims to be as comprehensive as possible, it is impossible to cover all of the content and scenarios that could come up in a test or real-life situation; therefore, for further background knowledge – not necessarily pertaining to the role of a nurse assistant – the learner should consult certified textbooks for medicine and nursing to assist them in defining areas where additional study is needed.

# Chapter 1: Foundations of Care

The foundational knowledge required of certified nursing assistants (CNAs) establishes the groundwork for safe, ethical, and compassionate care. This chapter provides a comprehensive overview of the core principles that will guide CNAs in their vital roles within the healthcare team. With this context, we will thoroughly explore the scope of practice, outlining permitted duties and prohibited activities. Legal and ethical considerations will also be discussed in depth, emphasizing healthcare policies, patient rights, documentation protocols, and liability risks. Mastering these essential concepts will equip CNA exam candidates with the theoretical framework and practical mindset needed to excel in providing person-centered care.

## Understanding the Role of the Nurse Aide

The role of the nurse aide, also known as a certified nursing assistant (CNA), is a vital part of the healthcare team. Though their duties may seem routine, CNAs provide the foundation of hands-on patient care that allows other medical staff to focus on more complex tasks. Understanding the scope, boundaries, and knowledge required to be an effective CNA is crucial for excelling in this position.

A CNA's responsibilities focus on assisting patients with activities of daily living (ADLs), such as bathing, dressing, using the restroom, eating, and moving around. CNAs help keep patients comfortable by repositioning them, providing skin care, taking vital signs, and reporting any concerns or changes as quickly as possible to the nursing staff. CNAs may also assist nurses with medical equipment and provide social interaction for patients. Strict boundaries are in place regarding what CNAs can and cannot do medically to ensure patient safety.

The scope of practice for a CNA is clearly defined by state regulations and healthcare facility policies. CNAs cannot administer medications, perform invasive procedures, or make independent judgments about care. Their role is centered on supporting nurses and doctors by carrying out basic care tasks. Exceeding their defined scope puts patients at risk and can result in disciplinary action.

To work effectively within their permitted duties, CNAs must possess certain core knowledge and skills. Required training covers topics like infection control, patients' rights, communication techniques, and safety procedures. On-the-job experience allows CNAs to become experts in properly moving patients, accurately measuring vitals, and efficiently assisting with ADLs. Soft skills like compassion and attention to detail also greatly impact a CNA's job performance.

## Legal Considerations for Nurse Aides

Certified nursing assistants have defined legal and ethical obligations that guide their practice. All actions must align with federal and state laws governing healthcare delivery, safeguarding patient rights, and defining parameters of professional conduct. From privacy protection and fraud/abuse prevention to avoiding negligence, CNAs must act lawfully, ethically, and in their patients' best interests. This section will examine key regulations, documentation standards, liability risks, and boundaries of legal practice that every nursing assistant must know. Mastery of these concepts will help CNAs feel empowered to deliver care with confidence and compassion.

### *HIPAA Privacy Rules*

The Health Insurance Portability and Accountability Act outlines patient privacy rights and prohibits the unauthorized disclosure of medical information by healthcare organizations and staff. CNAs must complete HIPAA training to gain authorization to access protected health details. However, they should only view essential data to fulfill their direct care duties and may not release records without permission. Privacy preservation is paramount.

### *Affordable Care Act and Changes to Reimbursement Models*

This expansive 2010 legislation increased health insurance coverage through measures like mandating state-run exchanges and enabling dependents up to age 26 to remain on parental policies. The ACA also initiated new models of value-based care and readmission reduction that shift Medicare reimbursement formulas toward quality outcomes rather than service quantity. CNAs support these changes through excellent care.

### *CMS Regulations for Nursing Homes*

CMS (Centers for Medicare and Medicaid Services) provides federal oversight for nursing facilities. CMS mandates standards for care, resident rights protections, facility staffing ratios, inspections, and survey protocols required for certification/recertification and participation in government payment programs. CNA practice must align with CMS rules.

### *OSHA Standards for Workplace Safety*

The Occupational Safety and Health Administration regulates exposure risks, injury prevention, and infection control in healthcare environments through right-to-know, hazard communication, and bloodborne pathogens standards. Proper PPE use, safe patient handling, ergonomics, and disposal procedures fall under OSHA purview to minimize the transmission of contaminants.

### Emerging Policies as Value-Based Care Models

Ongoing reforms continue shaping healthcare, such as new value-based funding models focused on enhancing patient outcomes while containing costs. CNAs positively impact this shift when trained in data gathering, preventive care, education, transitional support, and other interventions that improve community health and prove the value of coordinated teams.

### Right to Informed Consent and Shared Decision-Making

Patients have a right to receive clear information and ask questions before consenting to treatments or procedures. CNAs support this process by ensuring residents understand care plans and helping explain basics within their scope of practice respectfully, reporting concerns to nurses. Empowering them in care decisions is essential.

### Right to Privacy, Dignity, and Respect

Upholding patient privacy and dignity is central to ethical care. CNAs must protect the confidentiality of records, knock before entering rooms, speak softly near rooms, drape residents during care, and otherwise preserve modesty, comfort, and self-worth through careful, respectful interactions. Patients should retain their autonomy.

### Right to Freedom from Abuse, Neglect or Mistreatment

CNAs have a duty to shield patients from any form of abuse, neglect, or humiliation. This includes stopping inappropriate comments, reporting signs of physical harm or emotional distress, ensuring needs are met promptly, and promoting wellbeing through compassionate care. Protecting them is a moral obligation.

### Right to Access Records and Transparent Billing

Facilities must provide itemized billing statements upon request and share medical records with patients or their designated representatives appropriately. CNAs support transparency by never altering documentation and directing related inquiries to supervisors. Honesty and openness foster public trust.Right to File Grievances and Report Complaints

Nursing homes must present residents with their rights upon admission, including how to file formal grievances or complaints about perceived mistreatment, abuse, or substandard quality of care. CNAs assist by listening empathetically, documenting statements, and urging resolution through proper channels respectfully per policy.

### *Accurately Recording Vital Signs, Intake/Outputs, ADLs*

Clear, careful documentation is crucial. All CNA measurements, observations, and care actions must be recorded legibly in patients' charts. This includes vital signs, water/food intake and outputs, bodily fluid status, elimination patterns, ambulation distances, and ADL performance. Factually complete documentation provides essential medical-legal evidence.

### *Completing Forms, Charts, and Hourly Rounding Records*

In addition to notes, CNAs maintain records like admission logs, evaluation forms, daily skilled care flowsheets, meal intake percentages, hourly rounding sheets, restraint logs, and discharge documents. Completing forms legibly and fully demonstrates follow-through on care plans and regulations. Checklists help organize numerous responsibilities.

### *Following Proper Chain of Command for Concerns*

Reporting problems through proper channels is mandatory. CNAs immediately alert supervising nurses about risks or issues needing assessment, like injuries, conflicts, mistakes, safety hazards, and any patient statement suggesting abuse. A proper chain of command facilitates investigation, follow-up, and resolution.

### *Understanding Do-Not-Resuscitate Orders*

CNAs must know whether patients have advance directives like "do-not-resuscitate" (DNR) orders. DNRs only allow comfort care in the event of respiratory/cardiac arrest. CNAs help honor end-of-life wishes by knowing DNR status. They should assist during code situations as directed while respecting different choices.

## Ethical Principles in Healthcare

At its heart, healthcare is a moral obligation. The ethical delivery of services centers on respecting human dignity and the intrinsic worth of all patients. As direct caregivers, certified nursing assistants (CNAs) face ethical choices daily. Navigating dilemmas with compassion and integrity is paramount to patients and families, healthcare organizations, and CNAs themselves as moral agents.

## Autonomy and Respect for Persons

Patient autonomy is a cornerstone of ethical healthcare, where CNAs play a crucial role in facilitating self-determined decisions. This involves consulting residents about preferences, encouraging questions, and integrating their choices into care whenever possible. Honesty and transparency are key, as CNAs provide clear information to guide patients through care processes, promoting informed consent. Preserving privacy is paramount, with CNAs ensuring the confidentiality of personal information and maintaining dignity through respectful practices. Empowering patients through active listening and reminders of their rights underscores the commitment to autonomy.

## Beneficence and Promoting Good

Beneficence, the commitment to preventing harm and promoting wellbeing, drives CNAs to provide attentive care, disease prevention, and pain relief. CNAs judiciously balance risk and reward, ensuring proper use of therapies, reporting adverse reactions, and supporting shared decisions with healthcare professionals. Dedication to excellence defines ethical practice, with CNAs constantly refining technical skills, critical thinking, and compassion. Proactive measures, such as fall prevention, community health education, and encouraging engagement in life, demonstrate a commitment to fostering the holistic wellbeing of patients.

## Nonmaleficence and Avoiding Harm

Competence and prudence guide CNAs in preventing harm through proper body mechanics, infection control, and adherence to safety protocols. Continuous learning, training, and adherence to standards are essential in patient-focused care. Transparency in reporting issues or mistakes reflects integrity, contributing to a culture of safety. In situations requiring decisive response, CNAs may take direct action to stop preventable harm, such as intervening to prevent falls, reporting signs of potential harm or abuse, or clarifying medication-related miscommunications.

## Equal Treatment for All Patients

Justice in healthcare means that all people are equally deserving of safe, compassionate care regardless of identities, backgrounds, appearances, and abilities. CNAs demonstrate this by maintaining the same diligence and standards for every patient without judgment or prejudice. No one is more or less worthy.

### Fair Resource Allocation Without Discrimination

CNA attentiveness and time should be distributed impartially to meet each individual's care priorities. There must be no discrimination based on race, gender, religion, socioeconomic status, diagnosis, or any other protected classification. Needs come first in equitable care.

### Advocating for vulnerable or marginalized groups

Vulnerable patients depend on empathetic CNAs to speak up respectfully about unmet needs. CNAs promote justice and fairness by ensuring that those who cannot self-advocate fully still receive person-centered care in a judgment-free environment. Every life carries value.

### Reporting Illegal or Unethical Conduct

CNAs exhibit moral courage by holding team members and leadership accountable to legal/ethical standards if misconduct is witnessed or suspected. Violations must be reported properly to protect patients. Transparency about wrongdoing represents justice in action.

### Identifying and Analyzing Ethical Issues

Not every situation has an ideal solution. The first steps in ethical problem-solving are identifying the core issue and stakeholders involved, gathering pertinent facts, considering possible alternatives and their merits, and determining the least objectionable choice that honors duties. CNAs develop critical thinking to recognize dilemmas.

### Weighing Alternative Solutions and Consequences

Determining the best ethical path amidst competing concerns or priorities requires comparing options and projecting potential impacts. CNAs contemplate pros, cons, unintended consequences, and mitigation strategies. Input from nurses, doctors, and others informs well-reasoned resolutions.

### Collaborating with Team to Address Conflicts

Ethical issues rarely impact only one person. CNAs should engage peers, supervisors, clinicians, family if applicable, and the patient to address conflicts openly. Different viewpoints expand understanding and lead to decisions grounded in shared values. This fosters sustainable change.

### Documenting Objective Facts and Any Actions Taken

Thorough documentation helps track attempts to resolve concerns, completed follow-ups, and related statements. CNAs present only the factual timeline without judgmental language.

Subjective impressions belong in private exchanges with supervisors to determine if additional review or training is advisable.

## Reporting Unresolved Concerns Properly

If conflicts worsen despite interventions within CNA authority, the issue must ascend the proper chain of command to spur further action, starting with the charge nurse. CNAs provide accurate accounts of events to inform decision-making at higher levels if needed. They fulfill the ethical duty of voicing issues.

# Effective Communication in Healthcare

Communication is the foundation for safe, person-centered care. CNAs must develop excellent communication abilities spanning interpersonal rapport, active listening, clear self-expression, documentation skills, family updates, and coordinating within the interdisciplinary team. Mastering both verbal and nonverbal communication strategies enables CNAs to form therapeutic bonds with patients, gain crucial insights, provide comfort during distress, de-escalate tensions, educate effectively, and ensure continuity of care across settings. Communication mishaps, in contrast, readily lead to misunderstandings, loss of trust, gaps in care, conflicts, and poor outcomes.

## Active Listening and Focused Attention

Truly hearing others fosters understanding and trust. CNAs demonstrate active listening through undivided attention, maintaining eye contact at eye level, limiting interruptions, asking thoughtful questions, paraphrasing, validating emotions, and waiting thoughtfully before responding. These behaviors convey the message, "I hear you. I'm here."

## Clear Articulation Using Plain Language

To avoid ambiguity, CNAs speak clearly and directly but without condescension. Technical jargon is clarified or replaced with layperson's terms, reflecting an understanding of various literacy levels. Keeping vocabulary simple and pacing statements allows time for comprehension. Clarity prevents errors.

## Open-Ended Questioning and Empathy

Asking open-ended questions that go beyond yes/no responses encourages patients to elaborate on their experiences, concerns, goals, and objections. This guides decisions. CNAs also employ reflective statements like "This must be very difficult" to show empathy and support. Dialogue reveals unmet needs.

### Therapeutic Touch When Appropriate

With patient permission, therapeutic touch like holding a hand or a gentle hug provides nonverbal emotional support in difficult moments. However, social and cultural norms must guide the appropriate use of touch. CNAs remain sensitive to preferences, responding to cues from patients. Dialogue builds understanding.

### Cultural Differences in Spatial Boundaries

The degree of personal space varies between sociocultural groups. CNAs respect patients' potential preferences for more distance or limited touch, which are often subconscious boundaries. Getting permission before physical contact allows patients to feel comfortable. CNA adaptability prevents misunderstandings.

### Effective Clinical Documentation

High-quality documentation is accurate, objective, organized, legible, and timely. CNAs avoid editorializing. They use approved abbreviations and 24-hour clock time. Information flows logically from general to specific. Fact-finding with neutral language aids reader comprehension and demonstrates professional communication abilities.

### Organizing Notes Chronologically and Objectively

All events are recorded chronologically without subjective impressions to establish a factual timeline. CNAs avoid ambiguous phrasing by using clear vocabulary. Concrete details help paint an accurate picture: "Patient refused AM meds, stating 'They make me dizzy'" vs. vague charting like "Patient was noncompliant."

### Timely Completion of Forms, Reports and Records

Prompt documentation promotes coordination across shifts and disciplines. CNAs complete all charting within established time frames while details remain fresh. Late documentation appears sloppy. Flowsheets are updated each shift or hour as required. Timeliness is key for optimal continuity.

### Necessary Conciseness Balanced with Detail

Finding a balance between brevity and comprehensiveness presents a documentation challenge. Prioritizing the most essential information fosters conciseness. CNAs include enough focused detail to sufficiently convey the clinical picture and "tell the story" of care. Critical thinking guides relevance.

# Chapter 2: Safety Procedures

Safety is paramount in the healthcare environment, both for patients and healthcare workers. As a certified nursing assistant (CNA), it is crucial to understand and adhere to safety protocols to prevent injuries, control infections, and ensure overall wellbeing. This chapter provides an overview of essential safety procedures CNAs must follow, with a focus on infection control, emergency preparedness, and identifying and reporting abuse.

## Importance of Infection Control

Infection control is a central component of safety for CNAs. Proper techniques and consistent adherence to guidelines dramatically reduce the transmission of pathogens. From hand hygiene to utilizing barriers, CNAs serve as the frontline defense against the spread of infectious diseases.

### *Proper Hand Hygiene Techniques*

Hand hygiene forms the foundation of infection control. CNAs should wash their hands with soap and water when visibly soiled and use alcohol-based hand sanitizer if their hands are not visibly dirty. The six steps of proper hand washing are:

1) Wet hands and apply soap,
2) Lather soap covering all surfaces of hands for 15-20 seconds,
3) Rinse thoroughly under running water,
4) Dry hands with a disposable paper towel,
5) Use a towel to turn off the faucet,
6) Discard the paper towel.

CNAs should perform hand hygiene before and after all patient contact, after contact with contaminated surfaces, before donning gloves, after removing gloves, and before preparing or handling food.

### *Use of Personal Protective Equipment*

Personal protective equipment (PPE) creates a barrier against pathogens. PPE is usually made up of gloves, masks, gowns, goggles, as well as face shields. Gloves should be worn whenever there is potential contact with body fluids, blood, or contaminated surfaces. Gowns protect skin and clothing during procedures with the risk of splashes. Masks prevent droplet transmission when working near the mouth, nose, or respiratory equipment. Goggles or face shields guard the eyes from potential splashes during wound care or suctioning. PPE should be donned before patient interaction and removed slowly and properly before leaving the room.

## *Disinfection of Equipment*

Shared reusable equipment must be properly disinfected between patients to prevent cross-contamination. CNAs should wear gloves while disinfecting and allow full contact time for the disinfectant per manufacturer guidelines. Examples include using germicidal wipes on blood pressure cuffs, stethoscopes, lift slings and submerging bedpans in disinfectant. Careful disinfection protects patients from exposure to contagions through shared equipment.

## *Safe Injection Practices*

CNAs often administer insulin injections. Safe injection practices prevent the transmission of blood-borne pathogens between patients. CNAs should wear gloves, avoid recapping needles, immediately dispose of sharps in a puncture-proof container, disinfect reusable insulin pens between patients, and use single-use fingerstick devices. Following proper technique ensures injection safety.

## *Isolation Precautions*

Patients diagnosed with or suspected to have a contagious illness may be placed on isolation precautions. These could include contact, droplet, or airborne precautions. CNAs must strictly adhere to the appropriate PPE and hand hygiene procedures when interacting with an isolated patient. It is also essential to limit transport and ensure dedicated medical equipment. Isolation containment is vital to prevent the spread to other patients, visitors, and staff members.

## Emergency Protocols and First Aid

As frontline care providers, CNAs must know how to quickly and effectively respond to emergency situations to prevent further harm. Having strong knowledge of emergency protocols, first aid, and principles such as finding the scene safe will allow CNAs to act as key first responders.

## *Responding To Changes in Condition*

CNAs spend extensive time with patients and get to know their baseline status. Recognizing subtle changes from baseline could indicate an emerging emergency. For example, noting new pain, breathing changes, bleeding, or altered mental status requires promptly alerting the nurse. Early notification leads to rapid assessment and treatment, preventing further decline. Paying attention to alterations in condition often comes from developing a rapport with patients and learning their individual baseline. Subtle signs like facial grimacing, increased restlessness, or new onset agitation could signal the progression of illness. CNAs should trust their instincts if they sense something is amiss.

## Scene Safety

Before rushing to help in an emergency, CNAs must ensure the scene is safe. Dangers include live electrical lines, chemical spills, broken glass, and violent individuals. The first step is to pause and rapidly scan for potential hazards that could harm the CNA or others. Once the scene is confirmed safe, care can be provided. Attempting to intervene in an unsafe environment could result in injury or even death to the CNA and bystanders.

## Choking/Obstructed Airway

A blocked airway is a life-threatening emergency requiring immediate intervention. CNAs should be prepared to deliver back blows between the shoulder blades, abdominal thrusts, and manual finger sweeps for visible blockages. Calling for help while addressing choking is critical for patient survival. Recognizing the universal distress signal of clutching the throat and the inability to breathe or speak is fundamental for helping a choking patient. Quickly moving behind the patient to deliver five firm back blows between the shoulders can dislodge an obstruction. If unsuccessful, the Heimlich maneuver while standing behind the patient with arms encircling their waist can provide inward and upward abdominal thrusts to eject the blockage.

## Cardiopulmonary Resuscitation (CPR)

When someone goes into cardiac arrest, starting CPR can double or triple the survival odds. High-quality chest compressions at 100-120 bpm with minimal interruptions are key. CNAs should obtain certification and annual renewal in Basic Life Support (BLS) CPR to respond in an emergency. Using an automated external defibrillator (AED) and relief by rotating rescuers maintains effectiveness. Immediately beginning chest compressions can help oxygenated blood circulate to vital organs until emergency medical services arrive. Allowing full chest recoil between compressions and an adequate depth of at least 2 inches improves outcomes. Calling for the AED and using it quickly also increases the chances of successful defibrillation.

## Bleeding Emergencies

Bleeding emergencies require controlling blood loss through direct pressure, elevation, and pressure bandages. Applying tourniquets for limb bleeding and treating for shock are imperative.

CNAs should immediately report significant bleeding to activate emergency response teams for life-saving treatment. Realizing that quick action is required, direct pressure using clean dressings should be applied to visible bleeding sites. Elevating the injured area above the heart level helps slow blood flow. Tourniquets may be necessary for uncontrollable limb bleeding above pressure points. Monitoring for shock and immediately notifying emergency responders is key.

## Identifying and Reporting Abuse

CNAs are often closest to patients and, therefore, play a vital role in identifying and reporting any signs of potential abuse or neglect. Acting as a patient advocate means being constantly vigilant for subtle cues and promptly escalating concerns through proper channels to prevent further harm.

### Signs of Abuse

Possible indicators of abuse include unexplained injuries like bruises, burns, or fractures, withdrawal or fear around certain individuals, unusual weight loss, hygiene issues, untreated bedsores, or sexually transmitted infections. Behavior or mood changes could also signal abuse. CNAs should remain alert for clues while providing daily care. Unexplained lesions on areas not prone to accidental injury or markings in shapes suggesting human bite marks, grasp marks, or implements require careful documentation and reporting. Wariness around visitors or facility staff may also indicate troubling dynamics warranting discreet exploration.

### Reporting Procedures

First, promptly document objective observations only, avoiding opinions or accusations. Inform the immediate supervisor and follow the chain of command. Adhere to state mandatory reporting laws regarding reporting to authorities within specified timeframes if applicable. Provide all details to facilitate the investigation. Sticking to factual documentation without conjecture or confrontation is critical. Details like photographs of injuries with rulers for scale, verbatim statements or behaviors, and a timeline of pertinent observations over time can help investigators. Discretion prevents defensiveness as allegations are handled through appropriate channels.

### Maintaining Confidentiality

When escalating suspected abuse, CNAs should only share details with those directly involved in the investigation. Casual discussion with colleagues violates patient confidentiality and could impede official proceedings or place the patient at further risk. Information should be communicated discreetly through the proper channels only. Well-meaning gossip about suspicions may reach unintended ears and undermine efforts to protect the patient. All concerns should be shared privately with the charge nurse or appropriate manager to maintain the integrity of the investigative process.

## *Preventing Retaliation*

Fear of retaliation from an alleged abuser may make reporting difficult, but it must never prevent appropriate escalation. CNAs should report all concerns, knowing that regulations prohibit retaliation for good faith reporting. Advocacy to give at-risk patients a voice is a hallmark of compassionate care. Worries of backlash or reprisal may discourage reporting, but CNAs have a duty to speak up on behalf of vulnerable patients. Facility policies expressly forbid retaliation against any reporter.

# Chapter 3: Promoting Health and Wellness

A foundational component of quality patient care is promoting health and wellness through a holistic approach that addresses the physical, emotional, and mental wellbeing of patients. This chapter will provide an overview of key concepts relating to human anatomy, physiology, nutrition, hydration, and patient rights that CNAs must understand in order to properly care for patients and residents.

## Basics of Human Anatomy and Physiology

To perform their daily responsibilities safely and effectively, CNAs must have a solid grasp of basic human anatomy and physiology. Understanding how the body systems function and work together provides crucial context for various care tasks.

### Integumentary System

The integumentary system comprises the skin, hair, nails, and sweat glands. As the outermost layer of the body, the skin plays a major role in protecting internal structures from external factors like microbes, ultraviolet radiation, injuries, temperature extremes, and dehydration. Key functions include sensation, temperature regulation, vitamin D production, and excretion of water, salts, and wastes. CNA responsibilities involving the integumentary system include bathing patients, monitoring skin integrity, noting issues like rashes or pressure sores, and reporting abnormalities. When bathing patients, proper skin care techniques help maintain skin health. CNAs must carefully observe skin conditions and document any concerns, as many disorders manifest first on the skin. Providing appropriate skincare for each patient's age and condition promotes comfort and prevents complications.

### Musculoskeletal System

The musculoskeletal system includes bones, joints, muscles, tendons, and ligaments that provide shape, stability, movement, and protection. Bones produce blood cells and store minerals like calcium and phosphate. Joints enable mobility in areas where bones connect. Skeletal muscles attached to bones by tendons allow body movements and locomotion via contraction and relaxation. Cartilage provides cushioning between bones at joints. Ligaments join bones to form joints. Key CNA tasks tied to the musculoskeletal system involve moving and positioning residents, assisting with ambulation, lifting and transferring patients, and monitoring for limited mobility or paralysis. CNAs must use proper body mechanics during lifting and repositioning to avoid injury to patients and themselves. Noting pain, swelling, decreased mobility, and other abnormalities helps identify potential musculoskeletal issues needing medical attention.

## Circulatory System

The circulatory or cardiovascular system transports oxygen, nutrients, hormones, blood cells, and waste materials through the body via blood circulation. It includes the heart, blood and lymphatic vessels, and blood itself. The heart pumps blood through a network of arteries, arterioles, capillaries, venules, and veins. Blood delivers oxygen and nutrients to tissues while collecting waste like carbon dioxide to bring back to the lungs and kidneys for expulsion. Key tasks for CNAs involving the circulatory system include measuring pulse and blood pressure, reporting abnormalities, assisting with compression stockings, noting fluid retention, and watching for signs of stroke or heart attack. Monitoring pulse and blood pressure provides insight into cardiovascular health and early warning signs of problems. Proper application of compression stockings facilitates blood flow in the legs. Identifying sudden swelling could indicate congestive heart failure. Recognizing stroke and heart attack symptoms allows for rapid emergency care seeking.

## Respiratory System

The respiratory system includes not only the nose and lungs, but also the larynx, trachea, bronchi, and diaphragm. Its main function is facilitating gas exchange by bringing oxygen into the body and expelling carbon dioxide and other gaseous waste. During inhalation, the diaphragm and intercostal muscles contract to expand the lungs. Air enters the nose and passes the trachea and bronchi, ending in the alveoli. The alveolar membranes allow oxygen to enter blood vessels while carbon dioxide passes from the blood into the alveoli to be exhaled. CNA duties involving the respiratory system consist of taking respiratory rates, providing adequate ventilation and airway clearance, supporting oxygen therapy, and identifying issues like coughs or irregular breathing. Tracking respiratory rate gives insight into lung function. CNAs must ensure immobilized patients change position regularly to maximize air flow and prevent pneumonia. Understanding oxygen safety prevents fires. Noticing changes in breathing or coughing helps diagnose respiratory infections early.

## Nervous System

The nervous system regulates body functions via electrical nerve impulses and chemical signaling. It consists of the central and peripheral systems. The central includes the brain and spinal cord. The peripheral comprises the somatic and autonomic systems. The somatic involves voluntary movement and sensation. The autonomic controls involuntary functions like heart rate, breathing, digestion, and gland secretion. Nerves allow signals to travel from the brain and spinal cord to other body regions. CNA responsibilities tied to the nervous system include observing patients for stroke, seizures, head injuries, and paralysis while supporting activities like ambulation, transfers, and range of motion exercises. Signs of stroke include slurred speech, arm weakness, and facial drooping. Observing seizure activity assists in proper medication administration. Preventing head injury is vital, given the brain's fragility. Paralysis care aims to prevent pressure sores and contractures. The nervous system allows humans to sense and interact with the world, so damage can be debilitating.

## Endocrine System

The endocrine system encompasses glands and hormones that regulate various bodily functions. Major glands include the pituitary, thyroid, parathyroid, adrenal, pancreas, ovaries, and testes. These glands release hormones into the bloodstream to trigger organ responses. For instance, insulin from the pancreas regulates blood glucose levels. CNAs play a key role in assisting diabetic patients with insulin administration and blood sugar monitoring. They must know proper injection sites and techniques. Recording accurate intake and output information is important for electrolyte balance, given endocrine influences on thirst, urine output, and kidney function. CNAs also monitor for signs of hyperthyroidism, like rapid heart rate, hand tremors, and restlessness. Supporting endocrine health includes ensuring appropriate hormone replacement for deficiencies.

## Urinary System

The urinary system filters waste from the bloodstream and regulates water and electrolyte balance. The kidneys, ureters, bladder, and urethra are what make up the system. The kidneys remove wastes and excess fluid from the blood in order to produce urine. Urine is transported and stored until elimination thanks to the ureters, bladder, and urethra. Key CNA urinary care tasks involve monitoring fluid intake and output, assisting with toileting and incontinence management, identifying risks like infections, and supporting catheter and ostomy care. Adequate hydration prevents kidney problems and constipation. Catheter and ostomy care prevents infection while maintaining skin integrity. CNAs must recognize and report signs of urinary tract infections or kidney dysfunction like odor, cloudiness, discomfort, or reduced output. Supporting continence and managing episodes of incontinence preserve patient dignity while keeping skin dry.

## *Digestive System*

The digestive system processes food and liquid intake into usable nutrients and waste. Key components include the mouth, esophagus, stomach, intestines, rectum, anus, liver, gallbladder, and pancreas. Digestion begins mechanically in the mouth and then continues via enzyme action in the stomach, intestines, and pancreas. Absorption of nutrients and water mainly occurs in the small intestine. The liver produces bile to emulsify fats, while enzymes from the pancreas help digestion. The large intestine absorbs leftover water and compacts waste into the stool for elimination via the rectum and anus. CNA responsibilities tied to the digestive system involve maintaining appropriate nutrition and hydration, assisting with feeding and elimination, and monitoring issues like nausea, constipation, diarrhea, pain, swelling, or bleeding. CNAs help patients use the toilet or bedpans. Colostomy care ensures proper waste elimination. Reporting vomiting, abdominal distention, or bleeding helps identify gastrointestinal disorders.

## *Reproductive System*

The female and male reproductive systems facilitate human reproduction and sexual development. Female structures include the vagina, cervix, uterus, fallopian tubes, and ovaries. Male parts encompass the penis, scrotum, testicles, epididymis, vas deferens, seminal vesicles, ejaculatory duct, and prostate gland. Development begins in utero as chromosomes determine sex based on ovaries or testes formation. Puberty brings maturation of genitals and secondary sex characteristics driven by hormones. Menstruation signals female fertility. Key CNA tasks involve providing perineal care, assisting with hygiene during menstruation, supporting catheters or ostomies, observing for abnormal discharge, and ensuring privacy during care procedures. Perineal care keeps the genital region clean to prevent infections like yeast and urinary tract infections. CNAs must handle incontinence pads and assist with feminine hygiene products while preserving modesty.

## Understanding Residents' Rights

Upholding patient rights is a central ethical principle in healthcare. As frontline caregivers, CNAs play an integral role in ensuring patients and residents retain their autonomy, dignity, and individuality in care settings. Understanding essential rights and consistently demonstrating respect in interactions preserves personhood.

## Privacy and Confidentiality

Patients and residents have a right to privacy and confidentiality regarding their personal information and care. CNAs must keep medical records secure and refrain from sharing details publicly. Provide privacy during care tasks like bathing and toileting by utilizing curtains, closing doors, and speaking softly. Ask permission before sharing room details with visitors. Confirm identity prior to discussing care options on the phone. Disclose information only with appropriate staff to coordinate treatment plans. Upholding privacy preserves trust in caregiver relationships.

## Respect and Freedom from Abuse

Patients and residents have a right to considerate, respectful care and an abuse-free environment. Demonstrate respect through introductions, explanations, active listening, courteous language, cultural awareness, prompt care, and honoring preferences. Look for signs of potential neglect or abuse from caregivers or other residents and promptly report concerns through proper channels. Provide care gently—do not force participation if a patient refuses. Freedom from abuse encompasses physical, emotional, verbal, sexual, financial, and healthcare disparities. CNAs must help protect vulnerable populations.

## Information Sharing and Consent

Healthcare facilities must clearly communicate patient rights information in an understandable manner. CNAs play a role in reviewing rights upon admission. Patients have a right to accurate, timely information about their care, treatment options, and health outlook to make well-informed choices. Explain routines, procedures, and medications to patients while they give consent. Notify patients of risks, benefits, and alternatives. Honor medical decision-making documents like advance directives that outline wishes. Allow time for questions and clarify complex points. Informed consent promotes autonomy.

## Complaints and Grievances

Patients have a right to formally share care complaints without fear of reprisal. Facilities must provide clear grievance processes. CNAs should attempt conflict resolution verbally first when appropriate. Promptly relay unresolved complaints up the chain of command and to patient representatives. Facilitate problem-solving by listening neutrally and providing relevant details to nurse supervisors without blame. Comfort distressed patients while investigations occur. Handling grievances properly demonstrates responsiveness.

## Refusal of Treatment

Competent patients have the right to accept or refuse treatments or medications offered. CNAs must document and report all refusals to notify the care team. Do not attempt to pressure or persuade patients towards compliance—inform them of the risks associated with refusal and offer alternatives like reduced dosages. For severely impaired patients, follow advanced directives. In emergencies, life-saving measures take precedence until reviewed. While refusal can impact health, ultimately, it is the patient's decision.

## End-of-Life Choices

Terminally ill patients have specific care rights involving end-of-life choices. These include refusing treatments to prolong dying, selecting palliative therapeutic options for comfort, designating a surrogate decision maker, and establishing advance directives like living wills and do-not-resuscitate (DNR) orders that convey wishes. CNAs help uphold end-of-life choices by reviewing documents in charts, allowing patients to forgo interventions, adjusting care routines for comfort, providing spiritual resources, and notifying nurses of changes suggesting decline or actively dying status per facility policy. Honoring a patient's final wishes demonstrates compassion.

# Nutrition, Hydration, and Feeding Techniques

Proper nutrition and hydration are vital for supporting health and quality of life. CNAs play an integral role in assisting patients and residents with meeting nutritional needs by facilitating eating and drinking, utilizing special feeding techniques as required, monitoring intake and output, and identifying risks like dysphagia, dehydration, and malnutrition.

## Components Of Nutrition Care Plans

Facilities develop individualized nutrition care plans as part of the care planning process to meet patient's nutritional needs. CNAs must understand common components to properly assist residents at mealtimes. Plans outline diet orders and restrictions, such as regular, mechanic soft, diabetic, or thickened liquid. They specify the required food texture and liquid consistency. Plans identify the level of feeding assistance needed—independent, set-up help, intermittent prompting, or total assistance. Other elements include adaptive equipment like plate guards or built-up utensils, necessary positioning for feeding, and special instructions on pace or monitoring. Reviewing nutrition care plans prepares CNAs to provide aligned assistance.

## The Normal Swallow Process

Normal or healthy swallowing involves a coordinated sequence of nearly 100 muscles controlling the mouth, throat, and esophagus. Understanding this process provides context to recognize dysfunction. Oral preparation occurs as the tongue manipulates food, teeth chew, and saliva lubricates to form a bolus ready for swallowing. Oral transit involves tongue motion sweeping the bolus back towards the pharynx.

During pharyngeal transit, voluntary aspects transition to involuntary reflexes--larynx elevation, glottic closure, velar elevation, and upper esophageal sphincter opening enable bolus passage from mouth to esophagus without aspiration into airways. Esophageal transit through peristalsis brings the bolus to the stomach. Identifying impairments helps diagnose dysphagia.

## Dysphagia Signs and Symptoms

Dysphagia is a swallowing disorder that makes eating and drinking difficult or impossible. CNAs play a key role in identifying signs of possible dysphagia and reporting concerns. Oral phase issues include food remaining in the mouth, pocketing food in the cheeks, reduced chewing capability, drooling, or coughing/choking during meals.

Pharyngeal phase symptoms include gurgly vocal quality, nasal regurgitation, wheezing, or coughing after swallowing. Aspiration risks like recurrent pneumonia or changes in breathing patterns may occur.

Esophageal symptoms include feelings of obstruction, regurgitation, pain, or Valsalva maneuvers to bolster movement through the esophagus. Drooling, refusal to eat, weight loss, and malnutrition may develop. Early recognition facilitates intervention.

## Altered Diets and Appropriate Food Textures

Patients with chewing or swallowing difficulties often receive altered texture diets with food and liquid consistency modifications. CNAs must understand the terminology of meal plans. Regular diets have no limitations. Mechanical soft indicates ground or mashed foods like creamed potatoes or pureed carrots.

Thickened liquids are nectar, honey, or spoon thick. Low microbial or neutropenic diets exclude bacteria-prone foods. Low sodium, diabetic, renal, or cardiac diets control nutrients. CNAs must check food tray accuracy and offer appropriate encouragement and assistance during meals per training.

## Adaptive Devices for Feeding Assistance

Various adaptive devices help compensate for physical impairments that make self-feeding difficult. CNAs might incorporate aids like scoop bowls, plate guards, adapted handles, and cups with cut-out rims. Non-skid mats prevent dish slipping. Cups with attached straws or sipper lids allow for easier intake. For severe weakness, specialized feeding systems like automated arm supports may be needed. CNAs should obtain patient consent before implementing device use. Beginning with less invasive options helps maintain dignity. Multiple trials may be needed to optimize function.

## Proper Feeding Techniques

When assisting with patient meals, CNAs must utilize proper feeding techniques to maximize swallow safety, efficiency, and dignity. Key techniques include proper positioning, pacing, cueing, and environmental setup. Keep patients upright at 90 degrees to align the mouth, throat, and esophagus. Avoid distractions that could disrupt swallowing.

Offer small bites/sips and allow time to clear the mouth before advancing. Cue the person to swallow. Stop immediately if coughing or other signs of aspiration occur and report concerns. Employ clockwise feeding for visually impaired patients. Maintain eye contact and conversational cues to make mealtimes interactive. Proper techniques prevent complications.

## Importance of Rapport in Care Tasks

Positive rapport makes care tasks more pleasant for patients and easier for CNAs. Maintain eye contact when speaking or assisting with meals. Engage patients in light conversation by asking about favorite foods or special traditions. Be attentive to cues if chatter causes meal distraction. Offer encouragement for each bite or sip taken to affirm progress. Adjust your demeanor and pace to the patient's mood and energy level. When feeding is complete, thank individuals for allowing you to help them eat. Strong rapport increases cooperation.

## Snack and Meal Service Protocols

CNAs follow facility protocols when serving snacks and meals. Perform hand hygiene and gather the necessary supplies like plates, utensils, napkins, cups, and nourishment. Ensure tables are cleaned. Check meal orders. Retrieve trays delivered to the unit while items are still hot. Adjust table height for each patient. Place meal items within reach. Offer beverages first if desired. Encourage self-feeding if capable. Provide adaptive equipment as needed. End the meal with mouth care. Document percentage consumed or other issues. Handle leftovers according to policy. Following protocols prevents errors.

## Nourishments and Between Meal Offerings

Nourishment provides added calories between meals. CNAs prepare and serve items like snacks, crackers, pudding, ice cream, gelatin, nutrition supplements, or fortified beverages. Timing varies – mid-morning, mid-afternoon, and evening nourishments are typical. Serving nourishments helps boost nutritional intake, especially if meals are incomplete. Nourishment delivery also provides an opportunity to ensure adequate hydration between meals. CNAs make rounds with water, juice, or other beverages. Be alert for requests – the inability to communicate thirst directly makes proactive beverage offerings essential.

## Common Dietary Restrictions

Certain medical conditions and treatments warrant dietary restrictions. CNAs play a key role in understanding common diet limitations. Renal diets control electrolytes and minerals for kidney disease. Cardiac and low sodium diets reduce sodium to decrease fluid retention and heart strain. Thickened liquids help prevent aspiration. Gluten restrictions are fundamental for those who have Celiac disease. Diabetic diets balance carbohydrates. Protein limits may be needed for liver disease. Calorie maximums help with obesity. Dental soft diets ease chewing with tooth loss. Knowing common restrictions helps ensure nutritional needs are still met.

# Chapter 4: Essential Nursing Skills

Certified nursing assistants (CNAs) form the backbone of daily hands-on healthcare, providing basic care and assisting licensed nurses and other providers. To competently fulfill their critical role, CNAs must develop proficiency in a wide range of essential nursing skills. Mastering both fundamental knowledge and applied techniques allows CNAs to deliver safe, compassionate, and effective care.

## Recording Vital Signs: Procedures and Best Practices

One of the most important routine duties of a certified nursing assistant is accurately recording patients' vital signs. Vital signs—comprised of temperature, pulse, respiration, and blood pressure—provide crucial objective data about a person's physiological status. By regularly gathering and documenting a full set of vital signs, CNAs help provide critical insight into each patient's condition over time. This allows providers to detect improvements, deteriorations, or concerning trends and promptly intervene as needed.

To competently fulfill this central role, CNAs must demonstrate proper technique for obtaining vital signs and charting them correctly per nursing protocols.

### *Measuring Oral Temperature*

To correctly obtain an oral temperature, gather necessary supplies, including thermometer probe covers, a working digital thermometer with an intact probe, gloves, a timing device, paper, and a pen. Confirm that the thermometer is cleaned per manufacturer instructions. Carry out hand hygiene routine and put on clean gloves. Introduce yourself, explain the procedure, and verify patient consent. Ask the patient to remove any food, gum, or candy from their mouth. Place the new probe cover snugly over the thermometer tip. Turn on the thermometer unit and ensure it is reset from previous readings. Gently lift the patient's tongue with a tongue depressor and place a thermometer probe under the tongue on either side. Instruct patient to close mouth over the probe. Hold the thermometer in place under the tongue without biting down for full time per device recommendations, often 30-60 seconds. Time with watch/clock. When the thermometer beeps, signaling completion, remove the probe from their mouth. Read the temperature and immediately discard the used probe cover in a biohazard container. Wipe down the thermometer probe with an approved disinfectant wipe or solution. Record the temperature reading in the medical record, along with the current time and your initials. Notify the nurse of any abnormally high or low readings outside normal ranges. The oral temperature normal range is 97.8-99.1 degrees Fahrenheit. Remove gloves and perform hand hygiene. Thank the patient and ensure they are comfortable before leaving.

## *Measuring Radial Pulse*

The radial pulse in the wrist provides key data about a patient's heart rate and rhythm. To accurately measure radial pulse, gather equipment including a stethoscope, watch/timer, hand sanitizer, gloves, paper, and pen. Have the patient sit or lie with wrist and arm supported at heart level. Perform hand hygiene and don clean gloves. Explain the procedure to the patient. Position the patient's wrist so the palm faces up. Place your index and middle fingertips (not your thumb) over the inner wrist below the base of your thumb. Press gently until you feel the pulse. Look at the watch/timer and count the beats felt over 60 seconds. Also, assess rhythm (regular, irregular) and force (weak, normal, strong). Record measured pulse rate, rhythm, force, current time, on which wrist, and your initials in the medical record per policy. Compare reading to normal ranges for age. A typical adult radial pulse is 60-100 beats per minute. Report any readings outside normal ranges promptly. Remove gloves, perform hand hygiene, and ensure that the patient is comfortable before leaving.

Accuracy depends on proper fingertip placement on the radial artery away from the thumb and counting beats for a full 60 seconds. Abnormal rates, rhythms, or force require the nurse be notified.

## *Measuring Respiratory Rate*

A patient's respiratory or breathing rate over 60 seconds provides insight into lung function. To accurately measure, only a watch or timing device is needed. Stand where you can observe the patient's chest rise/fall. Without alerting the patient, watch chest/abdomen movement for one full minute to avoid altering the breathing rate. Count each complete respiration cycle (inhale and exhale) during the full 60-second period. Record measured respiratory rate, current time, and your initials in the medical record per policy. The typical adult respiratory rate is 12-20 breaths/minute. Rates under 12 or over 20 require prompt follow-up. Thank the patient and ensure their comfort before leaving.

Accuracy depends on covertly counting only full breath cycles for the complete 60-second duration. Abnormal high or low rates must be reported to the nurse ASAP as a potential medical emergency.

## Measuring Blood Pressure

Measuring blood pressure requires gathering equipment including a stethoscope, correctly sized arm blood pressure cuff, gauge/monitor, alcohol wipes, gloves, and recording form. Have the patient sit upright in a chair with their feet flat and arms resting on the surface at heart level. Expose the upper arm area. Clean their arm with an alcohol wipe.

Wrap the cuff snugly around the bare upper arm with an artery marker aligned over the brachial artery on the inner arm. Place the stethoscope bell on the brachial artery below the cuff. Inflate cuff to 30mmHg over typical systolic pressure. Close valve. Slowly release air from the cuff while listening for the first thump—systolic reading. Note that the point sound disappears—diastolic. Deflate the cuff fully. Record which arm is used, systolic/diastolic pressures, heart rate, time, and your initials. Repeat on the opposite arm and compare. Notify the nurse of any readings outside the normal range.

Typical and ideal reading is between 90/60mmHg and 120/80mmHg. High blood pressure requires prompt follow-up. Remove equipment, perform hand hygiene, and ensure the patient is comfortable before leaving.

Accurate measurement requires proper cuff sizing/placement and skillful use of the stethoscope. Compare left and right arm readings, which should be within 10mmHg. Abnormal readings must be reported immediately.

## Patterns and Documentation

Vital signs demonstrate important patterns. Elevated temperature may indicate infection. A heart rate over 100 beats per minute is tachycardia, while irregular rhythm may signal arrhythmia. Respiratory rate over 20 or under 12 requires rapid response. High or low blood pressure readings must also be addressed swiftly. Proper documentation is critical.

All vital sign measurements, times, and initials must be accurately recorded in the medical record per facility policy. Concerning abnormal readings or patterns, they should be reported to the nurse immediately.

## Infection Control

Strict infection control protects patients when obtaining vital signs. Proper hand hygiene before and after patient contact is essential. Gloves must be worn and changed between patients. All equipment should be cleaned and disinfected after each use. Used thermometer probe covers, and other disposable materials require immediate disposal in biohazard containers.

# Principles of Body Mechanics

Certified nursing assistants must manually move patients in beds and wheelchairs and assist with ambulation and transfers. The physical nature of the job places CNAs at high risk for back and muscle injuries. Utilizing proper body mechanics protects both patient and caregiver safety. Body mechanics refers to the coordinated effort of muscles, bones, and the nervous system that must be made in order to maintain balance, posture, and alignment during physical activity. Mastering basic mechanical principles and techniques will allow CNAs to perform manual handling tasks safely and effectively.

## *Centering And Balance*

Proper centering refers to keeping your body's center of gravity over the base of support to maintain balance. Feet should always be shoulder-width apart, with one foot slightly forward compared to the other. Bend knees and hips to keep the center of gravity low. Keep back straight. Look ahead, not down. Use leg muscles to bear weight, not the back. Moving feet to pivot or change direction is safer than twisting the back. Weight should be even on both feet when lifting/moving objects or patients.

## *Back Care Principles*

Use leg muscles and avoid bending from the waist to lift items. Keep back straight. Get close to the object with a wide, balanced stance before lifting. For heavy loads, keep the load close to the body and directly in front of you. Bend at hips and knees only to pick up the load. Hold the load close to the body while carrying it and avoid twisting or bending from the waist. Change direction using feet pivot steps. Kneel on one knee rather than bend over to access low objects. Use arm muscles rather than the back to push/pull objects.

## *Patient Transfers and Ambulation*

Use approved assistive devices such as gait belts, lifts, and walkers to reduce the risk of injury during transfers and walking. Keep back straight. Use legs and arm muscles to bear weight during patient lifts and transfers. Coordinate motions and communicate clearly with assistants and patients. When ambulating the patient, hold the gait belt firmly. Make sure you are wearing stable, non-slip footwear. Provide support on the affected side. Use gentle guidance, not pulling, along with verbal cues. Pivot and turn in the direction of the affected side to prevent across-body twisting during ambulation and transfers.

### *Bed Mobility and Positioning*

Raise the bed to waist level before repositioning, transferring, or making an occupied bed. Keep your back straight and bend your knees to move the patient. Stand close with a wide, balanced stance. Slide the patient using a draw sheet rather than lifting. Coordinate motions with helpers. When rolling the patient, tuck the side down and keep the body aligned. Avoid arm pulls and across-body twisting. Use approved lift devices for impaired patients. Keep back straight, and use leg muscles. Coordinate with helpers.

### *Body Mechanics in Daily Tasks*

Limit overhead reaching. Use step stools to avoid extra stretching. Slide objects along the countertop instead of carrying them. Sit close to the work area. Keep needed items within easy reach zone to avoid twisting and bending. Limit lifting heavy objects. Seek help and use dollies or carts for large/heavy items. Take micro-breaks to stand and stretch. Maintain optimal posture and joint alignment.

### *Safe Lifting Fundamentals*

Before any manual lift or transfer, assess the patient's condition and ability to assist. Explain the procedure and coordinate roles with helpers. Make sure you are wearing non-slip footwear. Remove obstacles and widen stance. Face the patient with feet shoulder-width apart, one slightly ahead. Get close to the load. Squat or kneel rather than bend. Hug the load close to the core and tighten the abdominal muscles. Lift straight up with legs, and keep back flat. Pivot feet to change direction. Coordinate with helpers.

## Care of the Environment and Patient Belongings

In addition to clinical care duties, CNAs play a central role in maintaining patient safety and well-being through the proper care of their environment and belongings. Tasks like bed-making, sanitizing surfaces, tidying rooms, storing personal items, and monitoring inventory must be performed skillfully and compassionately.

### *Bed Making*

Gather fresh linens and supplies. Lower bed, apply breaks. Raise the side rail opposite the working side. Loosen used linens, but leave the patient covered if they are still in the bed. Fold the edges of the fresh fitted sheet under the mattress. Anchor firmly. Place the flat sheet over the mattress. Center seam at middle of the bed. Allow at least 8 inches loose at the foot. Tuck loose ends under the mattress, so the sheet fits snugly. Miter corners. Avoid skin contact with dirty linens. Apply blanket/spread. Fold the top sheet down over the blanket. Replace pillowcase. Raise the head of the bed as needed.

## Patient Room Cleaning

Schedule cleaning when patients are out of the room. Gather approved cleaners and sanitizing supplies. Wash hands. Put on protective gear like gloves and gown as indicated. Follow protocols for high-touch surfaces. Clean floors from the furthest to the nearest exit. Change mop heads/buckets between isolation vs. non-isolation rooms. Remove soiled linens and trash promptly. Disinfect surfaces, including bed rails, tables, and controls. Allow to air dry. Clean spills or splatters immediately per policy. Report any pest issues promptly. Restock supplies. Remove protective gear carefully to avoid contamination. Wash hands after removing gloves.

## Daily and Terminal Cleaning

Daily cleaning involves quick tidying, sanitizing, removing trash, and restocking supplies between patients. Terminal cleaning is the deeper disinfection of the room after patient discharge in preparation for new occupancy. All horizontal surfaces are thoroughly washed with approved germicidal detergent. Allow air drying. Bathrooms/showers are scrubbed and disinfected. Toilet bowls are descaled. Drain traps are flushed. Floors are mopped with disinfectant. The ceiling vents are dusted. Walls are spot-cleaned if soiled.

Privacy curtains are changed, and the cubicle is disinfected. Used equipment is cleaned and returned. The room is restocked per policy. The nurse manager inspects and signs off before the room is reopened.

## Isolation Room Cleaning

Appropriate protective garb is worn to prevent the spread of pathogens in isolation areas. All supplies must remain inside the isolation room during cleaning. Special caution is used when handling contaminated linens and waste. Separate cleaning supplies and equipment are stored in the isolation anteroom.

These items do not leave isolation areas. When cleaning is complete, carefully remove protective garb and place it in a waste receptacle inside the anteroom. Scrub your hands before exiting. Signs remain on doors, identifying isolation precautions until the terminal cleaning process is fully inspected and approved.

## Responsible Item Storage

Patient valuables like eyeglasses, hearing aids, and dentures must be labeled and stored safely during care. Routinely document all patient valuables and belongings on intake and return on discharge. Securely store medications, equipment, linens, and supplies per policy. Use only designated storage areas. Lock wheeled equipment when not in use. Return devices to proper departments after use. Document inventory needs, such as lost or damaged items. Remove outdated or broken supplies promptly.

## Handling Personal Belongings

Always demonstrate respect for patient property. Avoid judging the value of items. Note and follow any cultural considerations regarding belongings. Ask permission before moving or handling items. Transport familiar objects with the patient when moving rooms or discharging to ease the transition. Inspect washable clothing and launder it according to any special instructions. Return all labeled items to the owner. Promptly report any lost or damaged property per facility policy. Secure replacement is the responsibility of the facility.

# Chapter 5: Personal Care Proficiencies

As a certified nursing assistant, many of your duties involve providing intimate personal care for patients. Assisting individuals with activities of daily living (ADLs) like bathing, grooming, dressing, and toileting is a central aspect of the CNA role. Performing these personal care tasks requires sensitivity, patience, and respect for human dignity.

## *Assisting with Activities of Daily Living (ADLs)*

Activities of daily living (ADLs) are the basic self-care tasks individuals perform regularly to live independently. ADLs include bathing, dressing, grooming, feeding, toileting, walking, transferring, and maintaining continence. CNAs play a central role in providing dignified assisted care for patients who are unable to fully carry out these activities themselves.

## *Bathing Patients*

Prepare area, water, and supplies at a safe temperature. Explain the procedure to the patient and respect privacy. Remove the gown, leaving the client covered. Use gentle motions. Bathe the upper body first, including the chest. Proceed to lower body/legs. Keep the patient warm. Wash face last and pat dry. Apply lotion while the skin is damp to hydrate. Avoid forceful rubbing of fragile skin. Help the patient dress in clean clothing and groom as tolerated after bathing. Prepare for rest.

## *Oral Hygiene and Denture Care*

Explain the procedure to the patient prior to providing oral care. Gather supplies: toothbrush, toothpaste, water, dentures. Gently brush natural teeth using small circles. Clean tongue and roof of mouth. Rinse thoroughly. For dentures, gently brush the device over the sink filled with water to avoid damage if dropped. Rinse well before placing it in the mouth.

If removing dentures, have a clean cup ready where you place the dentures after rinsing with clean, cold water and toothpaste. If desired, use a denture cleansing tablet in the cup filled with water. Then proceed to gently brush natural teeth and clean and rinse the mouth.

Ask if the patient would like lip balm or mouth moisturizer applied to prevent dryness.

## *Hair Care and Grooming*

Maintain patient's normal hairstyle as able. Ask preferences. Gather needed tools and products. For washing, tilt the head back in the sink or tub. Use a pitcher to wet hair and apply shampoo gently. Rinse fully. Pat dry. Apply conditioner or serum as requested. Comb out tangles slowly and carefully starting from the bottom. Shave patients as instructed using warm water and shaving cream. Rinse the razor frequently to prevent irritation. Trim fingernails and toenails carefully at the patient's request or as directed. Avoid cutting skin.

## Toileting and Incontinence Care

Ask the patient for normal elimination patterns and preferred toileting schedule. Assist patient to the bathroom regularly to avoid accidents. Watch for nonverbal signs of need, like agitation. If incontinent, check and change soiled garments/bedding promptly. Avoid over-hydrating before bed. Use a lifting device for transfer if needed. Clean the patient gently and thoroughly. Apply cream and dry pads/garments.

## Bed Mobility and Transfers

Raise the bed to a safe working level. Lower side rails on the movement side. Explain the plan for transfer to the patient. From supine to sitting: move knees up and help slowly turn onto the side. Lower legs down and help sit up using good body mechanics. For transfer to chair/commode: Position chair snugly to bedside with armrests lowered or removed. Use an approved transfer device. Stand with proper posture in front of the patient. Communicate and coordinate movements. Proceed slowly.

## Range of Motion and Positioning

Change patient position at least every 2 hours to avoid skin breakdown. Move up in bed and turn side to side and rearrange pillows. Perform gentle exercises daily as directed through range of motion to prevent contractures. Move joints slowly. Watch for signs of discomfort during movement, like grimacing. Stop immediately if any pain is voiced. Elevate the head of the bed to 30 degrees unless contraindicated to reduce pneumonia risk.

## Grooming and Hygiene Protocols

Proper grooming and hygiene are essential for a patient's comfort, health, and sense of self-worth. CNAs must skillfully attend to daily grooming needs, including nail care, shaving, oral hygiene, skincare, and more, while preserving patient dignity.

## Nail Care

Gather needed supplies: basin, warm water, mild soap, towel, nail clippers, file, and lotion. Explain the procedure to the patient and get permission before providing nail care. Immerse the patient's hands or feet in warm water for 5 minutes to soften nails. Dry thoroughly with a towel. Apply lotion and gently push back cuticles using a cotton-tipped applicator. Do not cut cuticles. Carefully trim nails straight across so tips extend just beyond fingers/toes. Use a nail file to gently smooth any rough edges. Clean under nails with cotton-tipped applicators soaked in warm, soapy water. Rinse and dry thoroughly; apply lotion.

## Shaving Patients

Determine patient preference for shaving: razor or electric, shaving cream/soap/gel, aftercare products. Prepare equipment and check for proper functioning. Draw a privacy curtain. Drape chest and lap with towels, and expose only the area being shaved. Apply warm, moist towels to the area for 2-3 minutes to soften skin and hair. Use circular motions. Apply shaving preparation product and shave in the direction of hair growth using short, gentle strokes, rinsing the razor frequently. Avoid pressing too firmly. Rinse the area well, dry thoroughly, and apply any aftershave or powder per the patient's request.

## Skin Care

Prevent dryness by applying lotion after bathing while the skin is still damp. Check for any red or raw areas daily. Avoid vigorous rubbing when drying skin—pat instead. Take special care around fragile areas like arms, heels, and elbows. Report any skin changes or concerns like rashes, redness, or breakdowns promptly to the nurse. Keep vulnerable skin protected. Adjust the bath routine if soap dries the skin. Use gentle cleansers and skin barrier ointments if directed.

## Proper Hand Hygiene

Hands are the key vector for infection transmission. Rigorously follow hand hygiene protocols. Wash hands with soap and water for 20 seconds before and after patient care. Use hand sanitizer if soap is unavailable. Scrub between fingers under nails. Rinse thoroughly and dry hands well on a clean towel or paper. Keep nails trimmed short. Avoid artificial nails. Report any breaks in the skin. Follow isolation procedure signs.

# Dressing, Undressing, and Comfort Measures

Certified nursing assistants routinely assist patients with dressing and undressing as well as providing other comfort measures. This involves competently helping don attire like shirts, pants, socks, shoes, gowns, robes, and briefs in a manner that respects privacy and maintains self-esteem.

CNAs must also be adept at utilizing devices and techniques to optimize patient ease and accessibility during care, including pillows, wedges, lift aids, and repositioning.

## Considerations for Dressing/Undressing

Always preserve patient privacy. Provide gown during procedures. Drape with linens to expose only the area being dressed/undressed. Explain each step to the patient and get permission beforehand. Watch for signs of fatigue or discomfort. Choose loose, comfortable clothing. Layer items for easy on/off. Adapt garments as needed for mobility devices or catheters. When undressing, inspect the skin. Report any concerns. Help patient wash as needed. Provide fresh garments.

## Shirts and Pants

Lay clothing flat on the bed. Roll pant legs up to slide over feet easily. Start with the weak or unaffected side first when possible. For shirts, insert the weak arm into the sleeve first, then slide the shirt overhead and onto the stronger arm. Use gentle guidance rather than force. When undressing, remove the strong arm sleeve first, then slide the shirt overhead and remove it from the weak arm. Avoid shoulder pulling. Help the patient stand to raise their pants. Check for a secure fit. Adjust as needed after the patient is seated again.

## Socks and Shoes

Select non-slip socks that are not too tight. Use sock aids if available to ease the process. Elevate feet and gather socks. Place socks over toes, heel, and up foot/ankle in one motion, smoothing the fabric up. When putting on shoes, always check the insides first and remove debris. Ensure the shoe is stable with appropriate heel height. Guide feet into shoes gently. Do not force. Tie/fasten as needed for a snug fit and support. Adjust several times once standing to verify comfort.

## Robes, Gowns, and Briefs

Warm robes or wraps prevent chill and preserve dignity when bedbound. Help the patient slide arms through sleeves. Tie securely and adjust as needed. Hospital gowns are tied in the back. Untie or lower to expose only areas needed for care access. Retie promptly, ensuring privacy after procedures. Check and change incontinence briefs at set intervals. Remove soiled briefs completely before skin cleansing and new brief application.

## Comfort Devices and Positions

Pillows support body alignment and prevent pressure. Position between knees, under head/neck, and beneath limbs as needed. Footboards provide stable footing when sitting up in bed. Trapeze bars allow patients to self-assist with transfers. Special mattresses like fluidized positioning beds mold to body contours for added comfort.

## Lifts And Transfers

Use approved transfer aids like transfer belts, sliding boards, and mechanical lifts to avoid injury when moving patients. Explain the need and process to the patient. Guide limbs one at a time. Keep body aligned during lift or transfer. For mechanical lift use, inspect the device function. Ensure the sling is properly positioned before lifting. Operate gently, avoiding sudden jerks. Have ambulation devices like canes ready at the bedside before assisting the patient to stand or transfer. Provide steadying assistance.

# Chapter 6: Mental and Social Care Needs

Mental and social care needs are at the heart of what CNAs do daily. It encompasses a wide spectrum of challenges, from addressing the psychological changes associated with aging to managing challenging behaviors and providing compassionate care to individuals with cognitive impairments and dementia.

To excel as a CNA, one must be equipped with the knowledge, skills, and empathy required to cater to the unique needs of each patient.

## Addressing Psychological Changes in Aging

As individuals age, they undergo a multitude of psychological changes that significantly impact their mental and emotional well-being. CNAs play a pivotal role in providing care and support to elderly patients, making it essential to comprehend these changes and how they can affect patient care.

### Understanding the Aging Process

Aging brings about a natural progression of changes, both physical and psychological. CNAs should have a foundational understanding of the normal aging process to differentiate between typical changes and potential signs of more serious psychological issues. This awareness helps in providing appropriate and tailored care.

### Emotional Needs of Elderly Patients

Recognizing and addressing the emotional needs of elderly patients is crucial. Many individuals may experience feelings of loneliness, loss, or a sense of diminished independence. CNAs can support emotional well-being by offering companionship, engaging in conversation, and fostering a positive and empathetic environment.

### Dealing with Grief and Loss

Grief and loss are common experiences for elderly individuals, whether related to the death of loved ones, declining health, or changes in living situations. CNAs can provide emotional support by actively listening, acknowledging feelings, and connecting individuals with additional support services, such as counseling or support groups.

## Empathy and Communication

Empathy plays a vital role in addressing psychological changes. CNAs should strive to understand the unique experiences and emotions of each elderly individual. Effective communication involves both verbal interactions and non-verbal cues, ensuring that patients feel heard and understood.

## Promoting Mental Well-Being

Creating an environment that promotes mental well-being is essential. This involves incorporating activities that stimulate cognitive function, providing opportunities for social interaction, and encouraging hobbies or interests that bring joy. CNAs can collaborate with other healthcare professionals to develop personalized care plans that address mental health needs.

## Emotional Intelligence in Care

Emotional intelligence enables CNAs to navigate the emotional complexities of aging with sensitivity. This includes recognizing and appropriately responding to emotional cues, adapting communication styles based on individual needs, and demonstrating empathy in challenging situations.

## The Impact of Stress on Aging Patients

Chronic stress can significantly impact an individual's mental and physical health. CNAs should be attuned to signs of stress in elderly patients and implement stress-reduction techniques. This may involve creating a calming environment, encouraging relaxation exercises, or facilitating activities that bring a sense of joy and peace.

## Dignity and Respect

Preserving the dignity and respect of elderly patients is fundamental. CNAs should approach care tasks with sensitivity, ensuring that individuals are actively involved in decisions about their care and are treated with the utmost respect, irrespective of their cognitive or physical abilities.

## Strategies for Managing Challenging Behaviors

Managing challenging behaviors in elderly patients is a crucial aspect of caregiving, necessitating effective strategies for Certified Nursing Assistants (CNAs).

Common challenging behaviors, including verbal or physical aggression, agitation, resistance to care, and wandering, may indicate underlying issues such as physical pain, discomfort, confusion, or unmet emotional needs.

When dealing with aggression, CNAs prioritize safety through de-escalation techniques, maintaining calmness, respectful distance, and non-confrontational language. Verbal aggression is approached with empathy and active listening to defuse situations effectively. For agitation and restlessness, redirection techniques involving positive or calming activities are employed.

Wandering, which poses safety risks, is addressed through collaborative efforts with the healthcare team, implementing environmental modifications, and utilizing technology for tracking.

Comprehensive documentation of challenging behaviors, including triggers and responses, is emphasized, providing invaluable insights for the healthcare team to assess patient needs and tailor care plans accordingly. Accurate reporting ensures the well-being of patients and facilitates the effective management of their behavioral challenges.

## Approaches to Cognitive Impairments and Dementia Care

Cognitive impairments are characterized by a decline in cognitive functions, including memory, reasoning, and language skills. Dementia, a common cognitive impairment, encompasses a range of disorders that affect memory and cognitive abilities. Some of the most well-known types of dementia include Alzheimer's disease and vascular dementia.

CNAs should be aware of the varying degrees of cognitive impairments and how they impact patients. The symptoms can manifest differently in each patient, and it is crucial to tailor care to meet their specific needs.

### *Dementia: A Comprehensive Overview*

Dementia is a progressive condition that affects not only memory but also judgment, problem-solving, and the ability to perform daily activities. It is vital for CNAs to have a comprehensive understanding of dementia to provide the best care possible. Key points to grasp include:

- Stages of Dementia: Dementia is often categorized into stages, from mild to severe. Each stage presents unique challenges and care needs.
- Behavioral Symptoms: Patients with dementia may exhibit various behavioral symptoms, including aggression, agitation, or wandering. These behaviors often stem from the patient's frustration or discomfort.
- Communication Difficulties: Dementia can impair a patient's ability to communicate effectively. CNAs should be skilled in non-verbal communication techniques, such as using visual cues and gestures to enhance understanding.

# Person-Centered Care

Person-centered care is an approach that, at the core of its care plan, places the individual being cared for. For patients with cognitive impairments, this means recognizing their unique history, preferences, and needs. CNAs should strive to establish a rapport with the patient, understanding their life story, likes, and dislikes.

By personalizing care, CNAs can enhance the patient's sense of identity and well-being. For instance, if a patient once enjoyed gardening, incorporating gardening-related activities or discussing past gardening experiences can be a source of comfort and engagement.

## *Creating A Supportive Environment*

The physical environment plays a crucial role in dementia care. CNAs should work with the healthcare team to create a safe and supportive setting for patients. This includes reducing environmental stressors, such as excessive noise or clutter, and implementing measures to prevent wandering or elopement.

Maintaining a consistent routine is also beneficial for patients with dementia. Familiarity can reduce anxiety and confusion. CNAs should ensure that daily activities, meals, and interactions occur at regular intervals.

## *Communication Strategies*

Effective communication is essential when caring for patients with cognitive impairments. CNAs should adapt their communication style to meet the patient's needs. Here are some key strategies:

- Use clear, simple language: Avoid complex sentences or medical jargon. Speak slowly and clearly.
- Non-verbal cues: Use facial expressions, gestures, and body language to convey information and emotions.
- Active listening: Pay close attention to the patient's verbal and non-verbal cues and respond with empathy.
- Validation therapy: Acknowledge the patient's feelings and emotions, even if they seem irrational. Validating their experience can reduce distress.
- Visual aids: Visual cues, such as picture cards or labeled objects, can help patients understand and participate in daily activities.

# Chapter 7: Basic Restorative Services

## Implementing Range of Motion Exercises

Range of motion (ROM) exercises are fundamental in maintaining and enhancing a patient's physical well-being. These exercises are designed to keep joints flexible, muscles strong, and the body agile. For patients who are confined to beds or wheelchairs or those who have limited mobility, CNAs often become the primary facilitators of ROM exercises.

## *Understanding Range of Motion Exercises*

ROM exercises are a set of activities that aim to maintain or improve the flexibility and mobility of a patient's joints. These exercises involve moving each joint through its full range of motion. There are two primary types of ROM exercises: active and passive.

### *Active ROM Exercises*

Active ROM exercises are performed by the patient without any assistance. In these exercises, the patient moves their joints and limbs through their full range of motion. These exercises are ideal for patients who have the ability to move independently. As a CNA, your role in active ROM exercises is to provide guidance motivation, and ensure that the patient performs them correctly.

### *Passive ROM Exercises*

Passive ROM exercises, on the other hand, are performed with the assistance of a caregiver, in this case, the CNA. Patients who are unable to move their limbs independently rely on passive ROM exercises to maintain joint flexibility. As a CNA, your role in passive ROM exercises involves gently moving the patient's joints for them, ensuring that each joint experiences its full range of motion. This not only helps in preventing joint contractures but also provides comfort to the patient by preventing stiffness.

## *CNA's Role in Implementing ROM Exercises*

As a CNA, you are at the forefront of implementing ROM exercises for patients.

Before initiating any ROM exercises, it is essential to assess the patient's range of motion and mobility limitations. This assessment helps you tailor the exercises to the patient's specific needs and capabilities. You are responsible for educating the patient on the importance of ROM exercises and motivating them to participate actively if possible. Providing clear and simple instructions can make the patient feel more comfortable with the exercises.

Safety is paramount during ROM exercises. CNAs must ensure that the exercises are performed without causing any pain or discomfort to the patient. Always communicate with the patient during the exercises to monitor their comfort level. For patients who require passive ROM exercises, CNAs play a crucial role in providing gentle assistance. You should move the patient's limbs through their full range of motion, ensuring that joints do not become stiff or fixed.

Keeping accurate records of the exercises performed, the patient's progress, and any issues or discomfort they may experience is essential. This documentation helps in tracking the effectiveness of the exercises and adjusting the plan as needed. Effective communication with the healthcare team, including nurses and physical therapists, is crucial. They can provide valuable input and adjustments to the ROM exercises as necessary.

## Ambulation and Use of Assistive Devices

Ambulation is a vital part of the restorative care that CNAs provide. Walking aids independence and well-being, so understanding proper techniques is important. This section outlines best practices in greater detail.

### *Gait Training Protocols*

As a CNA, you will likely be involved in gait training protocols under the direction of physical or occupational therapists. Proper form and supervision are key to avoiding injury while building strength. There are standard progressive methods commonly used.

Gait training often starts with posture education to encourage patients to stand and walk with correct alignment. Exercises may then focus on specific impaired areas, like balance with feet together, standing, or stepping with involved limbs. Advancement depends on the patient demonstrating stability and endurance with each skill.

Assistive devices are sometimes introduced early on for additional stability and confidence. Crutches or walkers allow patients to try standing safely and bear just enough weight to build tolerance gradually. Therapy teams closely monitor vital signs and fatigue levels to individualize walking programs appropriately.

Activities may progress to more functional tasks like walking in places with obstacles to navigate or up inclines. Marching in place, steps and other aerobic routines can also be incorporated. The goal is safe independence in all mobility skills needed for at-home activities of daily living. As such, transitions between positions and practice with braces or orthotics would be part of comprehensive gait re-education.

## Transfer Techniques

When assisting patients in and out of beds, chairs, vehicles, and more, CNAs must uphold safe practices. Before initiating transfers, assess for instructions from the nursing staff regarding health precautions or ergonomic adaptions.

Proper lift mechanics that avoid straining one's back are important. Good stance, bent knees, and using one's legs to do the work of lifting or lowering someone minimizes torque forces and prevents injuries. It's also wise for CNAs to seek help for heavier individuals rather than risk overexertion alone.

Additionally, transfers should be performed slowly and deliberately to ensure patient safety. Communicate directions clearly to maintain situational awareness while steadying or pivoting as one moves. Engage patient participation as able, having them shuffle feet cooperatively or push up with hands/arms for dynamic balance practice.

Be extremely mindful of complying with any doctors' activity restrictions, too. Some patients may have fragile bones prohibiting weight-bearing past a point, and others may have spinal limitations curbing certain motions. Nurses detail what is allowed to keep patients safe.

## Ambulation Aids

There are various assistive devices commonly incorporated into gait training, each suited to different mobility levels. As a CNA, it's important to understand proper usage to avoid mishaps.

Walkers provide stability for those with weakness who are able to bear weight partially on both legs. Patients should grip handles firmly and avoid leaning on the walker for more than 50% of their body weight. CNAs may need to prompt proper technique at first.

Canes work best for stronger individuals but still need an extra handhold to unload pressure on one leg. Patients are instructed to avoid any weight on the cane, keeping it mobile for balance each step. An improperly weighted cane could cause falls.

Wheelchairs allow full dependency for those non-weight-bearing for various reasons. Be mindful that some patients may still have arm function and desire to self-propel occasionally, so teaching basics like manual braking and turning assist in independent mobility.

Crutches are common for partial weight bearing on one leg and, like canes, are designed to keep that involved side unweighted. Swing-through motions with both crutches advancing in unison are key, along with proper fitting for overhead arm range and grip angles.

## Monitoring Vital Signs

Any exertion can affect bodies in Various Ways, so vigilant assessment is key during and after ambulation sessions. CNAs often check blood pressure, heart rate, oxygen saturation, and respiratory rates at a minimum.

Changes like elevations over a certain threshold or irregular beats could signal impending issues requiring a stop and re-evaluation. Documentation alerts the care team to possible intolerance developing from advancing levels of activity too quickly.

Prompt identification allows for timely intervention if dehydration, fatigue, postural hypotension, cardiac strain, or other troubling signs emerge. Continued assessment indicates safety to continue or when more rest is prudent before further gait challenges.

## Documenting Progress

Charting comprehensively on ambulation helps ensure continuity of programming between shifts. Include specifics like distances covered, need for breaks, use of assistive devices, and ability to navigate obstacles/turns.

Note observations about strength, balance, or coordination improvements. State tolerance and any persisting performance barriers requiring therapy focus. Flag positive behavior changes regarding engagement and willingness to walk independently.

Quantify functional progress weekly or monthly to recognize achievements. This data sharing establishes reliability for gait safety status updates with nurses, discharge planners, and home health referrals, together with vital records and a complete picture form.

## Offering Encouragement

Positive reinforcement is hugely motivating during gait training sessions. Celebrate efforts made and distances covered, no matter how small. Recognize progress toward locomotion milestones with genuine praise to boost confidence.

Allow patients to attempt walking without excess aids as strength permits them to feel accomplishment. Clapping or high-fives from CNAs after successful laps shows appreciation for the hard work put in during PT. This encouragement nurtures the drive to push limits.

Meanwhile, showing patience and understanding prevents discouragement if setbacks occur temporarily. Reassure recovery takes time, and your goal is to celebrate each small victory together along the way. An encouraging attitude keeps patients engaged.

When possible, allow curious peers watching from hallways to compliment neighbors putting in exertion. Social interaction can add therapeutic benefit and camaraderie for continued motivation during hospitalization or across outpatient treatments.

## *Working as a Team*

Coordinating with multiple members optimizes gait results. CNAs relay exercise logs and observations to physical or occupational therapists directing rehabilitation programs. Early signs needing adjustment are shared.

Dieticians ensure that protein-rich complimentary meal trays deliver fuel for muscle growth. Nurses provide medication reminders if prescriptions impact energy levels or functioning at all.

Activity coordinators may incorporate ambulation into scheduled group events. Therapeutic recreation opportunities could involve stimulating classes or sports fostering teamwork, memory, balance, and endurance together.

## *Additional Training Opportunities*

Some CNAs pursue supplementary certifications advancing expertise. Specialty courses teach techniques like Neuro-Developmental Treatment in handling patients recovering from neurological injuries.

Training in LSVT-BIG methodology optimizes loud, potent exercise, keeping patients intensely engaged physically and mentally post-stroke. Knowledge of sensory strategies engaging vision, balance, and proprioception enriches standard gait practices.

## Complication Prevention: Ulcers, Contractures, and More

As a CNA, preventing avoidable issues through best restorative practices yields substantial benefits. This section outlines strategies in greater depth to minimize complications jeopardizing health.

## *Pressure Ulcer Prevention*

Close skin checks are paramount, as well as inspecting bony areas prone to breakdown from prolonged pressure. Pay attention to the coccyx, heels, elbows, hips, shoulders, and ears particularly.

Any finding of non-blanchable redness requires immediate nursing notification. Early signs treated promptly may stop ulcer progression. Regularly shifting and repositioning non-ambulatory patients every 2 hours enables pressures to be relieved.

Padding techniques can displace weight from sensitive sites, too. Specialty overlays, gel cushions, booties, and handout pillows distribute forces evenly. Consistently implementing preventative measures becomes second nature with experience.

For higher-risk patients, a more rigorous Braden scale assessment, which assesses pressure sores, determines a tailored frequency of repositioning—possibly every hour or with each activity change. Nurses instruct specialized gowns, mattresses, or other durable medical equipment as needed.

## Nutritional Monitoring

Patients benefiting from restorative care require optimal fuel. Assess dietary intake records for sufficient protein, vitamins, minerals, and hydration contributing to healing.

Monitor appetites, chewing/swallowing issues, taste changes, or difficulties completing regular or pureed tray item that require notification. Address dislikes by suggesting alternate preferred choices.

Screen intolerance signs like nausea, diarrhea, constipation, or unintended weight changes needing intervention. Nutrition consultations address underfeeding risks compromising recovery. Together, the care team ensures dietary support.

## Environmental Modification

Make beds free of wrinkles or creases, not putting pressure on one spot too long. Smooth out sheets and straighten sleep surfaces each time patients are repositioned.

Ensure adequate lighting, comfortable temperatures between 70-80°F, and smoke-free air quality. Use non-irritating soaps and keep spaces clutter-free for safety. Hygiene cares similarly limit friction and shearing forces on the skin.

Regularly inspect mattress integrity and remove unnecessary tubes, minimizing entanglement risk. Documentation alerts maintenance if repairs are needed. Adapt little things impacting skin health and well-being.

## Prompt Wound Treatment

An assessing eye notices even minor wounds needing treatment elevation to heal properly without further breakdown. If any surrounding redness, swelling, or discharge exists, report observations to nurses. For existing ulcers or tears, check dressing conditions, drainage, and pain levels during shifts. Record measurements and describe appearances, noting improvements, declines, or changes requiring healthcare attention without delay. Prompt escalation aids recovery.

## *Bowel/Bladder Regularity*

Keeping elimination regimes consistent optimizes continence. Offer bathroom prompts during SHIFTS and maintain toileting logs, noting patterns and successes.

Notify nurses constipation signs so hydration or stool softeners can be adjusted. Incontinence products securely applied yet changed regularly also prevent skin maceration and worsening wound prognoses. Regularity establishes a routine.

## *Shared Vigilance*

Care conferences allow for the circulation of trenchant details between departments. Early complication indicators disclosed promptly invoke the quickest interdisciplinary responses. All hands work cooperatively for positive resolutions.

CNA discussions fill gaps between physician or therapy visits, ensuring consistent follow-through of prescribed preventative actions when patients are most vulnerable. This continuity safeguards wellness.

## *Patient Education*

Empowerment enhances participation in one's health maintenance. Explain in layperson terms what to watch out for, when to notify staff, hygiene best practices, and the importance of consistency in following discharge instructions.

Demonstrate proper lifting, pushing up from chairs, inspecting own backs, precautions in daily activities, and more to promote lifelong vigilance as people re-enter the community. Informed patients actively support their recoveries long-term.

# Chapter 8: Skills Evaluation Masterclass

## Preparing for the Practical Test

The practical test, also known as the skills evaluation, is a critical component of the CNA certification exam. It is the point where you must prove not only your theoretical understanding of nursing concepts but also your ability to apply these concepts in a real clinical setting. This part of the exam assesses your hands-on skills, judgment, communication, and, most importantly, your capacity to provide compassionate and patient-centered care.

To succeed in the practical test, you must first grasp its significance. It is not merely a formality; it is a reflection of your readiness to embark on a career in healthcare. Your performance during this evaluation will determine whether you are well-prepared to assist patients in their daily activities, ensure their comfort, and contribute to their overall well-being. To understand the gravity of the practical test is to understand its role in safeguarding patient safety and quality care.

### *Gaining Confidence Through Practice*

One of the most effective ways to prepare for the practical test is through practice. Practice allows you to build muscle memory, enhance your skills, and develop confidence in your abilities. Seek opportunities to practice essential skills and procedures. Joining a CNA training program or course is an ideal way to gain access to hands-on practice in a controlled, educational environment. These programs often provide simulated clinical experiences that mimic real-world healthcare settings.

However, do not limit your practice to the classroom or training program. Practice in various settings to adapt to different scenarios you might encounter during the exam. Volunteering at a healthcare facility or working as a caregiver under supervision can also provide invaluable hands-on experience. Remember, the more you practice, the more comfortable and confident you will become in performing the required skills during the practical test.

### *Understanding The Evaluation Process*

To excel in the practical test, you need a deep understanding of the evaluation process. This section will guide you through the key aspects of the evaluation, giving you a clear picture of what to expect. The evaluation process typically includes the following:

1. **Skill Stations:** The examiners set up skill stations where you are expected to perform specific skills or tasks. These stations are designed to assess your competence in various aspects of patient care, such as taking vital signs, providing personal care, and assisting with mobility.

2. **Demonstration:** You will be asked to demonstrate each skill, just as you would when caring for a real patient. Pay close attention to the examiner's instructions and follow them precisely. Keep in mind that communication and respect for the patient's dignity are essential components of the evaluation.

3. **Scoring:** Examiners will evaluate your performance based on specific criteria. Each step of the skill or procedure is graded, and you must meet a certain standard to pass. Familiarize yourself with the scoring rubric to understand how you will be assessed.

4. **Patient Simulation:** In some cases, the evaluation may involve working with a standardized patient or mannequin. This is done to simulate real patient-care scenarios and assess your ability to adapt to different situations.

5. **Time Limit:** There is usually a time limit for each skill station. You must complete the required tasks within the allotted time, which varies depending on the skill being tested.

By understanding the evaluation process, you can better prepare for what lies ahead, reducing anxiety and ensuring a smoother experience during the practical test.

## *Preparing Your Mindset*

Success in the practical test is not solely about your technical skills. Your mindset and attitude play a significant role in your performance. Approach the practical test with a positive and focused mindset. Believe in your abilities and remind yourself that you have acquired the necessary skills and knowledge through your training.

Managing test anxiety is crucial for peak performance. Implement relaxation techniques, such as deep breathing or visualization, to calm your nerves. Additionally, maintain a growth mindset. Understand that mistakes and failures are opportunities for learning and improvement. Embrace challenges and setbacks as part of your journey toward becoming a proficient CNA.

## *Organizing Your Resources*

Before the practical test, you must ensure that you have all the necessary resources and materials organized. This includes:

1. **Uniform:** Wear the appropriate uniform, usually scrubs, with your identification badge.

2. **Tools and Equipment:** Check and double-check that you have all the tools and equipment you will need to perform the required skills. This may include a blood pressure cuff, stethoscope, thermometer, gloves, and any other relevant items.

3. **Identification:** Bring your identification documents, which may include a driver's license or government-issued ID, as well as your examination admission ticket.

4. **Confidence:** Carry with you the confidence you have built through practice and preparation. A positive and confident attitude can greatly impact your performance.

5. **Notebook and Pen:** It is a good idea to have a small notebook and pen for taking notes, if necessary. However, you should check with your testing facility's rules regarding the use of such materials.

By meticulously organizing your resources, you will minimize stress on the day of the practical test and ensure that you are fully prepared to demonstrate your skills.

## *Test-Day Etiquette and Conduct*

The way you conduct yourself on the day of the practical test can influence your overall performance. Here are some key etiquettes and conduct tips to keep in mind:

1. **Arrive Early:** Aim to arrive at the testing site well before the scheduled start time. This will give you ample time to complete any registration or administrative procedures.

2. **Professional Appearance:** Dress professionally in your uniform and ensure you are well-groomed. This demonstrates your commitment to the role of a CNA.

3. **Communication:** When interacting with examiners, patients (if applicable), and fellow candidates, maintain clear and respectful communication. Show empathy and kindness, just as you would when caring for patients in a real healthcare setting.

4. **Follow Instructions:** Pay close attention to instructions provided by examiners and adhere to their guidance during the evaluation. This demonstrates your ability to follow directions, an essential skill for a CNA.

5. **Time Management:** Keep an eye on the time and manage it wisely during each skill station. Prioritize tasks, and if you find yourself running short on time, communicate this to the examiner and make an effort to complete as much as possible within the allotted time.

By understanding and implementing these principles of test-day etiquette and conduct, you will present yourself as a capable and professional CNA candidate, which can positively influence the evaluation process.

## Demonstrating Core Skills: Step-by-Step Breakdown

The practical portion of the CNA certification exam is designed to assess your ability to perform essential skills in a healthcare setting. In this section, we will break down some of the core skills you may be tested on, offering a step-by-step guide to help you navigate each skill with confidence and precision.

Each skill is a critical aspect of patient care, and your ability to perform them correctly and efficiently is essential to becoming a successful CNA. The skills you will learn here are not only vital for the exam but also for your future role as a healthcare professional. As you read through the following subsections, keep in mind that practice, practice, and more practice are key to mastering these skills.

### *Hand Hygiene*

One of the fundamental skills you'll be evaluated on is proper hand hygiene. Hand hygiene is a cornerstone of infection control in healthcare settings. To perform this skill correctly:

1. **Step 1 - Gather Supplies:** Before approaching the patient, gather the necessary supplies, including soap, running water, and paper towels.
2. **Step 2 - Wet Hands:** Turn on the water and wet your hands thoroughly. Make sure to use warm, not hot, water.
3. **Step 3 - Apply Soap:** Apply a sufficient amount of soap to your hands.
4. **Step 4 - Create Friction:** Rub your hands together vigorously, making sure to lather all surfaces, including the backs of your hands, between your fingers, and under your nails. This should take at least 20 seconds.
5. **Step 5 - Rinse Thoroughly:** Rinse your hands thoroughly, ensuring that all soap is removed.
6. **Step 6 - Dry Hands:** Use a clean, dry paper towel to dry your hands, starting at the fingertips and moving up the wrists.
7. **Step 7 - Turn Off Faucet:** Use the paper towel to turn off the faucet to avoid recontaminating your hands.

Proper hand hygiene is a skill that must be executed meticulously to prevent the spread of infections in healthcare settings. Always follow facility-specific protocols, and be mindful of the time needed for effective handwashing.

## Assisting with Activities of Daily Living (ADLs)

Assisting patients with their Activities of Daily Living (ADLs) is a core responsibility of a CNA. This skill set encompasses various tasks, such as bathing, dressing, grooming, and toileting. To assist a patient with bathing, follow these steps:

1. **Step 1 - Gather Supplies:** Collect all the necessary items, including soap, washcloths, towels, and any assistive devices the patient requires.
2. **Step 2 - Prepare the Environment:** Ensure the room is warm, the water temperature is comfortable, and maintain the patient's privacy.
3. **Step 3 - Explain the Procedure:** Communicate with the patient, explaining what you are going to do and ensuring you have their consent.
4. **Step 4 - Assist with Undressing:** Help the patient undress, providing assistance as needed.
5. **Step 5 - Ensure Safety:** Make sure the patient is secure in the shower or bath, and be prepared to offer support if they need it.
6. **Step 6 - Provide Personal Space:** Respect the patient's dignity and privacy while assisting with bathing. Only expose the areas necessary for washing.
7. **Step 7 - Thoroughly Clean:** Gently wash the patient using a washcloth and soap, paying particular attention to areas that require special care.
8. **Step 8 - Rinse and Dry:** Ensure all soap is rinsed off, and then help the patient dry thoroughly.
9. **Step 9 - Assist with Dressing:** Help the patient get dressed, maintaining their comfort and dignity.
10. **Step 10 - Final Checks:** Ensure the patient is comfortable, their environment is clean and safe, and their needs are met.

The key to assisting with ADLs is to provide compassionate, respectful care while maintaining the patient's autonomy and dignity.

## Vital Signs Measurement

Measuring vital signs accurately is another essential skill for a CNA. Vital signs include temperature, pulse, respiration rate, and blood pressure. To perform this skill correctly:

1. **Step 1 - Prepare Equipment:** Gather the necessary equipment, including a thermometer, blood pressure cuff, stethoscope, and a clock or watch.

2. **Step 2 - Explain the Procedure:** Communicate with the patient, explaining that you will be measuring their vital signs.

3. **Step 3 - Measure Temperature:** If measuring temperature, follow the manufacturer's instructions for the thermometer being used. Typically, this involves placing the thermometer under the patient's tongue, in the ear, or on the forehead.

4. **Step 4 - Measure Pulse:** Locate the patient's pulse (usually on the wrist or neck) and count the beats for 60 seconds.

5. **Step 5 - Measure Respiration Rate:** Observe the rise and fall of the patient's chest or abdomen, counting the number of breaths for 60 seconds.

6. **Step 6 - Measure Blood Pressure:** Apply the blood pressure cuff as instructed, using the stethoscope to listen for the pulse sounds. Inflate the cuff and slowly release the pressure while listening for the systolic and diastolic blood pressure readings.

7. **Step 7 - Record and Report:** Record the vital sign measurements accurately and report any unusual findings to the appropriate healthcare professional.

Measuring vital signs accurately is crucial for detecting any changes in a patient's health status. As a CNA, you must be proficient in this skill to provide the best care possible.

## *Assisting with Mobility*

Assisting patients with mobility is a common task for CNAs, especially those working in long-term care facilities. Patients may need help with moving from their bed to a chair, walking, or using assistive devices. To assist a patient with mobility:

1. **Step 1 - Prepare the Environment:** Ensure the patient's surroundings are clear of obstacles and hazards.

2. **Step 2 - Explain the Procedure:** Communicate with the patient, explaining the plan for assisting with mobility. Obtain their consent and cooperation.

3. **Step 3 - Use Proper Body Mechanics:** Bend your knees, keep your back straight, and use your legs, not your back, to lift. Maintain good posture to prevent injury to yourself or the patient.

4. **Step 4 - Use Assistive Devices:** If applicable, use mobility aids such as a gait belt or walker to support the patient's movement.

5. **Step 5 - Encourage the Patient:** Encourage the patient to assist as much as possible, according to their capabilities.

6. **Step 6 - Provide Steady Support:** Support the patient as they move, maintaining their balance and ensuring their safety.

7. **Step 7 - Secure the Patient:** Assist the patient in sitting or lying down safely and comfortably, and ensure they have any needed items within reach.

Maintaining proper body mechanics and prioritizing patient safety is essential when assisting with mobility. By mastering this skill, you'll be able to enhance the quality of life for those in your care.

## *Infection Control*

Infection control is a skill that every healthcare professional must master to ensure patient safety and prevent the spread of diseases. To effectively control infections:

1. **Step 1 - Hand Hygiene:** Always begin by performing proper hand hygiene as described in Section 8.2.2.

2. **Step 2 - Use Personal Protective Equipment (PPE):** Wear appropriate PPE, including gloves, gowns, masks, and eye protection, as needed, based on the specific task and patient condition.

3. **Step 3 - Isolation Precautions:** If the patient is on isolation precautions due to a known or suspected infectious disease, follow the facility's protocols for entering and exiting their room and using the appropriate PPE.

4. **Step 4 - Disinfection and Sterilization:** Understand the difference between disinfection and sterilization and use the appropriate method to clean and disinfect equipment and surfaces. Follow the manufacturer's instructions for disinfectants and sterilization equipment.

5. **Step 5 - Safe Waste Disposal:** Dispose of waste materials, especially biohazardous materials, in accordance with facility guidelines and regulations.

6. **Step 6 - Patient and Environment Hygiene:** Assist the patient with maintaining personal hygiene, such as bathing and toileting, to prevent the spread of infection. Also, ensure the patient's environment is clean and safe.

7. **Step 7 - Prevent Cross-Contamination:** Be mindful of your movements and avoid cross-contamination between patients. Change gloves and perform hand hygiene between patient interactions.

## Expert Tips and Common Pitfalls

Demonstrating care beyond mere competence is paramount in effective caregiving. As a CNA, your ability to provide a caring and reassuring presence outweighs technical skills. Simple gestures like smiling, making eye contact, and addressing residents respectfully by title or name set a positive tone. Reading and mirroring body language enhances comfort while introducing yourself and explaining procedures in a calm voice fosters a sense of ease. Paying attention to non-verbal cues, adapting to residents' or patients' comfort levels, and building rapport through conversation contribute to personalized and compassionate care.

Attention to safety precautions is non-negotiable. Clear communication, involvement of residents in decision-making, and checking safety equipment ensure a secure environment. Before initiating any procedure, explain it in simple terms, obtain consent, and confirm the resident's comfort. Double-checking surroundings for hazards and maintaining vigilance during activities like ambulation are crucial. Documenting and reporting safety issues promptly demonstrates a commitment to resident safety and well-being.

Remaining calm under pressure is a vital skill. Deep breathing and maintaining composure during stressful situations showcase poise. Admitting mistakes gracefully, correcting them respectfully, and learning from experiences contribute to professional growth. Double-checking work for accuracy, especially during moments of stress, prevents errors. Thoroughly scanning workspaces, confirming equipment placements, and narrating your thought process during tasks serve as self-check mechanisms, ensuring precision in caregiving until the very end.

# Chapter 9: Exam Strategy and Test-Taking Skills

Passing the Certified Nursing Assistant (CNA) exam is the crucial final step in securing your license and launching your career in healthcare. While the exam certainly tests your knowledge and practical abilities, it also evaluates your test-taking skills. Developing strategies to navigate the unique challenges of a high-stakes licensing exam can make the difference between passing and failing. This chapter provides insights and techniques to help you optimize your performance when exam day arrives.

## Navigating Multiple Choice Questions: Tips and Tricks

Multiple choice questions are the predominant format on the CNA written exam, so it is crucial to understand key strategies for tackling them effectively. First, read the question stem carefully, underlining or circling any terms that stand out as significant. The question stem provides context that will guide your approach to selecting the correct answer. Next, read through all of the choices before selecting one answer. This gives you a comprehensive view of the options and allows you to make comparisons between them. As you consider each choice, determine if it directly addresses the question posed in the stem.

Be wary of options that seem only vaguely related or use absolute words like "never" or "always" - while they may sometimes be correct, absolutes are rarely the best answer. Eliminate any choices that are clearly wrong based on your knowledge. If uncertain between two answers, try plugging each back into the original question to see which choice responds to it most precisely.

Do not overthink questions and change your response unless you misread something initially - your first choice is typically the right one. Also, do not get hung up on any single tough question. Make your best-educated guess and move on. You can return to tricky questions later if there is time.

The key is maintaining focus and confidence, trusting in your preparation, and applying these strategies thoughtfully across all questions. Avoid common mistakes such as choosing an answer that seems plausible but does not fully address the question. With practice, these techniques will help maximize your multiple-choice success.

## Time Management Techniques

The CNA exam must be completed within the mandated time, so utilizing savvy time management techniques is imperative. First, always scan the entire test at the outset to get a sense of the topics covered, the number of questions, and their difficulty level. This will allow you to budget your time accordingly. Move through the sections where you feel most confident first, answering those questions thoroughly to accrue points while your energy is highest.

For more challenging sections, start with the easiest questions to build momentum. Leave more time-consuming questions for later and simply mark them to revisit if time allows. With about 10 minutes left, quickly fill in any totally random guesses on unanswered questions, as there is no penalty for guessing. Working at a steady, controlled pace is key - moving too fast breeds carelessness, but working too slowly risks leaving questions unanswered. Jot down any key facts, formulas, or acronyms during breaks to boost recall efficiency when returning to questions. Practicing timed mock exams will hone your ability to pace yourself accurately. Managing your time strategically can mean the difference between a passing and failing score.

## Overcoming Test Anxiety

It is normal to feel some stress before or during an important exam, but excessive anxiety can actually impede your performance. If you struggle with serious test anxiety, using relaxation techniques in the weeks beforehand can help diffuse nerves come test day. When studying, take regular short breaks to practice deep breathing, meditation, or calming exercises like mindful coloring.

Ensure you get adequate sleep and nutrition leading up to the exam so you feel focused and energized. Upon sitting for the test, begin by taking some deep centering breaths. Affirm that you are well-prepared and focus only on the question at hand, detaching from how others around you seem to be progressing.

Anxiety often stems from negative self-talk and fear of failure - counter this by consciously replacing doubtful thoughts with empowering ones. Remind yourself that you know the material and have trained for this. If you get flustered by a tricky question, pause and recenter yourself before proceeding.

Persevering through nerves takes practice - each test will boost your confidence. With the right preparation and mindset, anxiety need not be an obstacle to your success. You've got this!

# Chapter 10: Comprehensive Practice Questions and Scenarios

Passing the Certified Nursing Assistant (CNA) exam requires thorough preparation and extensive practice. This chapter provides a robust set of sample questions and scenarios across all exam content areas to assess your knowledge and hone your test-taking skills. With 4 practice tests and a variety of hands-on skill scenarios, it offers a simulation of the actual testing experience to build confidence and identify areas needing further review.

## Exam Test Training

This section contains 4 sample exams, each with detailed explanations. These tests allow readers to experience the format, style, and level of difficulty of the actual CNA exam while assessing their knowledge. Depending on the state in which you will take the exam, the exam will be between 60 and 70 questions. We are offering 82 questions that have been divided into 4 groups to do at your convenience. If you want to do them all together or a little at a time, that is up to you!

# EXAM 1

1) **Which of the following describes the proper handwashing technique?**

A. Wet hands, apply soap, rub hands together for at least 20 seconds, rinse hands under running water, dry hands with a paper towel, and turn off the faucet with a paper towel.

B. Wet hands, apply soap, rub hands together for 10 seconds, rinse hands under running water, dry hands with a cloth towel, and turn off the faucet with bare hands.

C. Wet hands, apply soap, rub hands together for 30 seconds, rinse hands under running water, leave hands wet, and turn off the faucet with bare hands.

D. Wet hands, apply soap, rub hands together for 15 seconds, rinse hands under running water, leave hands wet, and turn off the faucet with a paper towel.

2) **Which of the following statements accurately describes the purpose of giving a bed bath to a patient?**

A. To clean the patient and inspect the skin

B. To provide passive range of motion exercises

C. To offer the patient a chance to get out of bed

D. To reposition the patient in bed

3) **Which of the following is an example of an open-ended question?**

A. Are you feeling sad today?

B. Do you have any concerns you want to discuss?

C. Do you need anything for pain right now?

D. Have you taken your medication this morning?

4) **Which of the following medications is considered a blood thinner?**

A. Ibuprofen

B. Warfarin

C. Lisinopril

D. Amlodipine

5) **Which of the following statements best describes the purpose of external catheter use in male patients?**

A. To promote continence through consistent urine output monitoring

B. To prevent urinary tract infections

C. To reduce the risk of falls associated with frequent urination

D. To provide comfort and convenience compared to urinary catheters

6) **Which of the following blood pressure readings is considered hypertensive?**

A. 122/78 mm Hg

B. 132/72 mm Hg

C. 148/92 mm Hg

D. 108/74 mm Hg

7) **Which of the following statements is true about a range of motion exercises?**

A. Passive range of motion exercises are preferred to active.

B. They should always be performed quickly with force.

C. They should be discontinued if the patient voices discomfort.

D. Lower extremities get a greater benefit than upper extremities.

8) **Which of the following is a right of a patient when receiving healthcare?**

A. To have a family member present for all procedures

B. To view his medical records at any time

C. To be transferred to another room if requested

D. To receive care without discrimination

9) **The S in the SAMPLE pneumonic for patient history stands for:**

A. Symptoms

B. Safety

C. Speech

D. Signs

10) **Which of the following statements reflects ethical practice by a CNA?**

A. Calling out sick from work to attend a social event

B. Discussing details of care for one patient with another patient

C. Adjusting an oxygen flow rate without proper training

D. Reporting unsafe practices in the workplace to a supervisor

11) **Which of the following is a right of healthcare workers under OSHA?**

A. Right to adequate personal protective equipment

B. Right to smoke in designated break areas

C. Right to receive overtime pay for shifts over 40 hours

D. Right to have weekends off if desired

12) *Which of the following symptoms warrants immediate notification of a nurse?*

A. The patient reports feeling nauseous after eating

B. Patient rates pain at 8 out of 10

C. The patient has a blood pressure of 138/100 mmHg

D. The patient has warm, reddened skin over their sacrum

13) *The nursing assistant notices a patient suddenly experiencing slurred speech. What is the most appropriate action?*

A. Ask the patient if they have been drinking alcohol

B. Lower the head of the patient's bed

C. Notify the nurse immediately

D. Bring the patient a glass of water

14) *Which of the following situations reflects the proper use of restraints for a patient?*

A. Restraining a combative patient without an order from the physician

B. Using a restraint to limit a patient's movement without frequently monitoring

C. Applying a restraint that is ill-fitting for the patient

D. Implementing a restraint to safely prevent a patient from falling

15) *Which of the following is an example of a breach of confidentiality?*

A. Discussing test results with other staff involved in the patient's care

B. Leaving patient charts open where others walking by can view them

C. Disclosing a patient's diagnosis to their spouse upon request

D. Reporting safety risks noted during care to the nursing supervisor

16) *The nursing assistant is asked to take a verbal prescription order over the phone from the physician and administer the medication immediately. What is the correct action?*

A. Take the verbal order, administer the medication, and chart it after

B. Ask the physician to come to the patient care unit and write the order

C. Wait to receive the written order before administering the medication

D. Have the nurse take the verbal order from the physician instead

17) **Which of the following statements best describes the purpose of flexing the hips and knees of a bedridden patient?**

A. To strengthen the hip and leg muscles through active exercise

B. To prevent contractures and maintain joint mobility

C. To prepare the patient for getting out of bed and ambulating

D. To assess neurological status and sensation in the lower extremities

18) **Which of the following is classified as a rights-based ethical concern in healthcare?**

A. Medical errors and negligence

B. Improper documentation

C. Patient autonomy

D. Poor communication

19) **Which of the following actions reflects caring in nursing assistant practice?**

A. Helping a patient wash up before a physical exam

B. Debating treatment options with the nursing supervisor

C. Assisting with a bed linen change while on break

D. Calling in sick when not feeling well before a shift

20) **Which of the following characteristics are important for a nursing assistant when communicating with patients?**

A. Patience, understanding, active listening

B. Speed, multitasking, focused interactions

C. Professional appearance, proper posture, eye contact

D. Confidence, sense of humor, casual language

# EXAM 2

*1)* **Which of the following best describes the purpose of a urine output record?**

A. To provide an accurate intake and output balance

B. To monitor kidney function and hydration status

C. To identify the need for urinary catheters

D. To determine the stage of continence training

*2)* **Which of the following statements is true about aspiration?**

A. It involves the discharge of fluids from the respiratory tract.

B. It typically occurs in patients with normal gag reflexes.

C. Thick liquids like nectar are less risky than thin liquids.

D. Keeping the patient in a semi-Fowler's position helps prevent it.

*3)* **A nursing assistant observes a licensed practical nurse (LPN) performing skilled procedures. Which action should the nursing assistant take?**

A. Remind the LPN that the procedure should only be done by an RN

B. Offer to assist the LPN if needed

C. Notify the nursing supervisor of the LPN's actions

D. Document the LPN's completion of the skilled procedure

*4)* **The nursing assistant enters the room of a patient who appears unresponsive. After verifying unresponsiveness, what is the next appropriate action?**

A. Call the patient's name while gently shaking their shoulder.

B. Administer ammonia inhalant and check for a response

C. Perform abdominal thrusts in case of airway obstruction

D. Immediately contact emergency medical services

*5)* **Which of the following is an appropriate intervention to prevent depression in a long-term care patient?**

A. Encouraging participation in group activities

B. Assisting with ADLs to increase dependence

C. Assigning seating in the same location daily

D. Providing medications on a PRN basis

6) *Where would a patient with dementia be residing if they have no other particular health issues?*

A. In a hospital

B. In a nursing home

C. In an Assisted Living Facility (ALF)

D. In a hospice

7) *Which of the following actions reflects ethical practice by a nursing assistant?*

A. Posting pictures of care provided to patients online without permission

B. Performing skills not competently trained for when told by the nurse

C. Reporting unsafe activities in the workplace to patient advocacy groups

D. Voicing disagreement with a care plan change directly to the patient

8) *Mr. Smith yells at the nursing assistant after being assisted to the bathroom. Which of the following is the best response?*

A. Telling Mr. Smith it is the nursing assistant's job to help him

B. Calmly asking if Mr. Smith needed more time to use the toilet himself

C. Informing Mr. Smith, he will now require a Foley catheter

D. Notifying the charge nurse about Mr. Smith's behavior

9) *Which of the following statements is true regarding the range of motion for a patient on bedrest?*

A. Active range of motion is preferred to passive

B. Lower extremities receive greater benefits than upper extremities

C. It should be performed quickly with exaggerated movements

D. Joints are taken just beyond the point of resistance

10) *Which of the following statements best describes the purpose of setting up the food tray at chin level for a patient?*

A. Allows patient to exercise arms by lifting fork to mouth

B. Provides an ergonomic position to prevent strain

C. Creates proper table manners and etiquette

D. Facilitates self-feeding with minimal assistance

11) **Which of the following statements reflects legal and ethical practice when communicating with other healthcare providers about patients?**

A. Disclosing information only to those directly involved in a patient's care

B. Allowing providers to access records without patient permission

C. Waiting to discuss care until the provider introduces themselves

D. Withholding opinions about the performance or competence of others

12) **Which of the following would be inappropriate to include in the handoff report between nursing assistants at shift change?**

A. Details of care provided during the previous shift

B. Updates on patient mental health status

C. Recommendations for improving patient care

D. Vital signs and other recorded measurements

13) **Which of the following actions demonstrates ethical and legal accountability for nursing assistants?**

A. Performing skills that have not been formally delegated

B. Reporting risks noted in the environment right away

C. Documenting care under the signature of a supervising nurse

D. Consulting with the nursing assistant team before contacting providers

14) **Which of the following characteristics is essential for nursing assistants to demonstrate during patient care?**

A. Studiousness

B. Stoicism

C. Empathy

D. Talkativeness

15) **Which of the following findings in the bedbound patient indicates a pressure ulcer is beginning to develop?**

A. Complaints of pain over bony prominences

B. Localized edema on one side

C. Reddened areas that blanch with pressure

D. Small blistered areas of intact skin

16) *A nursing assistant finds an unresponsive resident with vomit in the mouth. Which action should the nursing assistant take next?*

A. Clear the airway of vomit immediately.

B. Begin chest compressions and send for an AED

C. Start rescue breathing using a resuscitation mask

D. Check pulse and call 911 before intervening

17) *Which of the following statements most accurately reflects the nursing assistant's role in providing oral hygiene?*

A. Inspecting oral cavity tissue and structures

B. Obtaining dental orders from providers

C. Suctioning secretions from the oropharynx

D. Brushing/flossing teeth and cleaning dentures

18) *Which of the following situations reflects ethical decision-making as a nursing assistant?*

A. Calling in sick due to being tired from partying the previous night

B. Telling a confused patient it is lunchtime when it is actually afternoon

C. Prioritizing care based on which patients are most pleasant

D. Calling a nurse to perform tracheostomy suctioning in an emergency

19) *Which of the following reflects ethical practice when a nursing assistant observes unethical behavior by a coworker?*

A. Discuss the issue only with other nursing assistants

B. Report the problem directly to the state licensing board

C. Share concerns privately with the charge nurse

D. Place an anonymous report in the compliance box

20) *A nursing assistant notices a lapse in care provided by an LPN. Which response demonstrates ethical responsibility?*

A. Tell the LPNs they need to improve their job performance

B. Report the LPN's action to the nurse manager

C. Discuss the lapse with the nursing assistant team for input

D. Document details of the lapse in the chart for corrective action

# EXAM 3

1) **Which of the following demonstrates ethical responsibility by a nursing assistant when an error is made in patient care?**

   A. Documenting the lapse fully before the end of the shift

   B. Telling the patient an emergency came up suddenly

   C. Discussing the mistake only with the charge nurse

   D. Pretending the error did not happen

2) **The nursing assistant notices a coworker posted patient information online. What should be the next action?**

   A. Report the breach to the charge nurse immediately.

   B. Delete the online post to prevent further sharing.

   C. Discuss posting concerns privately with the coworker.

   D. Forward a screenshot anonymously to the administration.

3) **The nursing assistant finds an unlabeled syringe of medication left unattended. What should the nursing assistant do next?**

   A. Ask the nursing staff who it belongs to and return it

   B. Dispose of the medication in a sharp container

   C. Locate the order and try to identify the medication

   D. Put the syringe in a safe place until there is time to investigate

4) **Which of the following constitutes unethical practice by a nursing assistant regarding documentation?**

   A. Recording objective, factual information about care provided

   B. Noting concerns about possible neglect by family members

   C. Adding missing details to another staff member's charting

   D. Documenting assessments performed by a licensed nurse

5) **Which of the following actions by the nursing assistant reflects ethical practice when there is disagreement about patient care?**

   A. Voicing opposition directly to the patient

   B. Refusing to participate in the planned care

   C. Discussing concerns privately with the nurse

   D. Sabotaging implementation of the care plan

6) **A nursing assistant notices a fellow nursing assistant posted protected patient photos online. What is the next appropriate step?**

   A. Report the violation to the charge nurse immediately.

   B. Request the nurse manager speak to the nursing assistant privately.

   C. Delete the photos to prevent further breach of privacy.

   D. Comment on the post encouraging the removal of the photos.

7) **Which of the following statements reflects ethical practice by a nursing assistant who made a medication error?**

   A. Discussing the mistake only with the charge nurse

   B. Pretending the error did not happen

   C. Telling the patient a pharmacy mix-up occurred

   D. Acknowledging the error fully in the medical record

8) **A nursing assistant is asked to care for a resident of a race she feels biased towards. What action reflects ethical practice?**

   A. Request reassignment to a different resident for comfort

   B. Provide care, recognizing personal biases as unethical

   C. Do minimal care for the resident to avoid proximity

   D. Petition the nursing home to respect preferences in assignments

9) **A nursing assistant is asked to sign a document stating that a wound dressing was changed. However, the nursing assistant did not actually change the dressing. Which response is most ethical?**

   A. Sign the document because the dressing likely was changed

   B. Ask who changed the dressing before deciding to sign

   C. Agree to sign now and clarify the facts later

   D. Refuse to sign for care not personally provided

10) **A nursing assistant notices a coworker taking photographs of residents on a personal cell phone. What is the priority action of the nursing assistant?**

   A. Report the violation immediately to the charge nurse.

   B. Encourage coworkers to delete photos to prevent sharing.

   C. Review photo policies and secure phone with a coworker.

   D. Notify the state health department compliance line.

11) **Which of the following actions reflects ethical practice by a nursing assistant who observes resident abuse?**

A. Ask the resident if abuse is occurring before reporting.

B. Take photographs to document injuries for investigation.

C. Report suspicions immediately to Adult Protective Services.

D. Discuss concerns privately first with the charge nurse.

12) **The nursing assistant notices a coworker performing a procedure incorrectly. Which response is most appropriate?**

A. Stop the coworker and correct their technique right away

B. Report the unsafe practice to the nursing supervisor

C. Ask where the coworker learned the questionable technique

D. After, discuss the correct procedure with the coworker

13) **When a patient has difficulty swallowing because of a physical condition and requires thickened liquids, what is this condition called?**

A. Tachycardia

B. Atrophy

C. Dysphagia

D. Infection

14) **Which of the following constitutes unethical practice by a nursing assistant?**

A. Reporting unsafe patient ratios impacting care

B. Performing skills that have not been formally delegated

C. Sharing opinions about policy changes during the break

D. Documenting late entries marked with the current date

15) **A nursing assistant notices a nurse colleague acting impaired by intoxication at work. Which action is most appropriate?**

A. Approach and express concern about the nurse's condition.

B. Report the suspected impairment privately to the charge nurse.

C. Photograph the nurse's behavior to document for administration.

D. Remove the nurse from patient care responsibilities immediately.

16) **Which of the following actions reflects a nursing assistant's duty to maintain professional boundaries?**

A. Avoiding discussion of personal issues with residents

B. Declining friend requests from residents' families online

C. Refusing to assist with dressing changes after hours

D. Preventing a resident from independently operating a wheelchair

17) **A nursing assistant finds a resident on the floor complaining of hip pain after a fall. What should the nursing assistant do first?**

A. Try to lift the resident back into bed

B. Check for medical alert bracelets or signs of injury

C. Ask what happened and if the resident tried to get up alone

D. Move the resident just off the floor and onto a pillow

18) **Which of the following actions reflects caring by a nursing assistant toward a dying resident?**

A. Attempting to feed the residents if they refuse meals

B. Distracting the resident with funny stories and laughter

C. Sitting with the resident without judgment or goals

D. Reminding the resident of happy moments throughout their life

19) **Which of the following situations requires nursing assistants to breach patient confidentiality?**

A. Releasing records to an insurance company with patient permission

B. Reporting evidence of abuse, neglect, or domestic violence

C. Disclosing health information to law enforcement without permission

D. Notifying the health department about reportable diseases

20) **Which of the following actions reflects ethical behavior by a nursing assistant who made an error in patient care?**

A. Discussing the mistake only with nursing supervisors

B. Pretending the error did not happen

C. Telling the patient an emergency came up suddenly

D. Apologizing and discussing how to prevent future errors

# EXAM 4

1) **Which of the following special care needs would be most appropriate for a nursing assistant to assist with?**

   A. Inserting an indwelling urinary catheter

   B. Administering chemotherapy medications

   C. Changing central line dressings

   D. Testing capillary blood glucose levels

2) **Which of the following actions reflects ethical practice as a nursing assistant?**

   A. Posting about a patient's care on social media

   B. Performing a new procedure learned online

   C. Refusing to provide care based on personal beliefs

   D. Reporting unsafe practices by coworkers

3) **Which of the following is true regarding passive range of motion exercises?**

   A. They should be performed quickly with bouncing movements at the joint's end.

   B. They increase muscle tone and strength.

   C. They are performed by the nursing assistant on the patient.

   D. They are more beneficial than the active range of motion.

4) **The nursing assistant enters a room and finds an elderly resident on the floor next to the bed. What should be the nursing assistant's first action?**

   A. Help the resident back into bed immediately

   B. Assess the resident for any injuries that require treatment

   C. Use the call light to summon help moving the resident

   D. Ask the residents if they are hurt and what happened

5) **Which of the following types of legal documents can nursing assistants request from residents?**

   A. Power of attorney for healthcare

   B. Do not resuscitate orders

   C. Guardianship order

   D. Advance healthcare directives

6) **Which of the following statements accurately reflects the nursing assistant's role in feeding patients?**

A. Thickening liquids to the proper consistency

B. Obtaining diet orders from providers

C. Assessing the swallowing status of patients

D. Providing partial assistance to residents as needed

7) **Which of the following actions by a nursing assistant reflects ethical practice?**

A. Repeating a rumor about the unit manager

B. Posting pictures of a resident to social media without permission

C. Performing skills not adequately trained for when told by a nurse

D. Reporting safety concerns about new medical equipment

8) **Which of the following statements is true about purulent wound drainage?**

A. It indicates normal healing.

B. It should be reported to the nurse immediately.

C. It should be cleaned with peroxide and alcohol.

D. It requires wearing a mask, gloves, and a sterile gown.

9) **Which of the following actions reflects ethical decision-making as a nursing assistant?**

A. Calling in sick to attend a concert despite inadequate staffing.

B. Performing tracheostomy suctioning to help a nurse finish quicker.

C. Refusing to care for an abusive patient based on personal biases.

D. Reporting safety issues with new equipment despite peer pressure.

10) **The nursing assistant notices a diabetic patient's breath smells strongly of acetone. Which action is most appropriate?**

A. Give the patient orange juice right away.

B. Report it immediately to the nurse.

C. Check the patient's blood glucose level.

D. Document it on the patient's nutritional intake record.

**11) A nursing assistant finds a resident face down on the floor. After ensuring scene safety, what should be the next action?**

A. Rush to turn the resident face up to open the airway

B. Check for responsiveness, pulse, and breathing

C. Leave the resident stabilized while seeking assistance

D. Assess if any injuries require immediate treatment

**12) Which of the following constitutes an invasion of privacy for a patient?**

A. A nursing assistant enters a room without knocking.

B. Hospital staff viewing medical records as required for care.

C. Security cameras in hallways for safety.

D. Routine charting about the care provided.

**13) Which of the following tasks could a nursing assistant appropriately accept from a licensed practical nurse (LPN)?**

A. Administering oxygen therapy

B. Changing sterile wound dressings

C. Inserting a nasogastric tube

D. Applying warm compresses to legs

**14) When a dementia patient does not remember who you are and is agitated, what do you do?**

A. Talk to them calmly, introduce yourself and explain how you are going to assist them.

B. Call their family to inform them.

C. Remind them that they should remember you since you help them everyday.

D. Downplay the situation and insist that they will remember.

**15) Which patient should you attend to first?**

A. A patient who requires a bed bath

B. A patient who requires a bedpan

C. A patient who is hungry

D. A patient who is cold

16) **If a physician asks a nursing assistant to change the wound dressing of a patient, what should the assistant do?**

A. Change the dressing carefully after proper hand hygiene and putting on gloves

B. Call the nurse to change the dressing.

C. Tell the physician it is their responsibility.

D. Remind the physician that it is not in their scope and to ask a nurse to do it.

17) **When a patient has been bedridden for a longer period of time, it is important to assist the patient in ambulation because they probably have developed:**

A. Muscle atrophy

B. Ostomy

C. Dysphagia

D. Stroke

18) **If a patient is choking, a nursing assistant is trained to do which of the following as a response?**

A. CPR

B. Tracheostomy suction

C. Heimlich Maneuver

D. Put the patient on the ground

19) **Where would nursing assistants NOT typically work?**

A. At a dentist' office

B. At a hospice

C. At a hospital

D. At an adult day care center

20) **Which of the following actions reflects ethical practice by a nursing assistant who made a medication error?**

A. Discussing the mistake only with the charge nurse

B. Pretending the error did not happen

C. Telling the patient a pharmacy mix-up occurred

D. Acknowledging the error fully in the medical record

21) **Which of the following actions constitutes ethical practice by a nursing assistant?**

A.  Calling in sick in order to attend a party

B.  Telling a resident their roommate said unkind things about them

C.  Prioritizing care based on which residents give better gifts

D.  Reporting unsafe, incompetent, or unethical conduct of coworkers

22) **How should a nursing assistant assist a patient with dressing?**

A.  Give all the clothes to the patient at once and watch them dress themselves.

B.  If there is a weaker side, start from the stronger side.

C.  Dress quickly to avoid colds.

D.  Disregard the patient's care plan if the weather allows it.

# EXAM 1 - CORRECT ANSWERS

1) A

Explanation: Proper handwashing technique involves wetting hands, applying soap, rubbing hands together vigorously for at least 20 seconds, rinsing under running water, drying hands thoroughly with a paper towel, and turning off the faucet using the paper towel to avoid recontamination. This helps remove pathogens from the skin's surface.

2) A

Explanation: The purpose of giving a bed bath to a patient is to clean the skin through washing and rinsing while also inspecting the skin for any abnormalities. This helps maintain patient hygiene and detect skin issues early on.

3) B

Explanation: Open-ended questions cannot be answered with a simple yes/no, and encourage the patient to provide more detail. "Do you have any concerns you want to discuss?" is open-ended, allowing the patient to voice concerns. The other options can be answered with yes/no.

4) B

Explanation: Warfarin is a commonly prescribed anticoagulant, also known as a blood thinner. It works by inhibiting the formation of blood clots. Ibuprofen is an NSAID pain reliever, lisinopril is an ACE inhibitor used for hypertension, and amlodipine is a calcium channel blocker also used for hypertension.

5) D

Explanation: External catheters in males are used to provide comfort and convenience by allowing urine to drain into a collection bag, eliminating the need for bedpans or frequent trips to the bathroom. It does not necessarily promote continence or reduce infections or falls.

6) C

Explanation: Blood pressure is considered hypertensive when it measures at or above 140/90 mm Hg, which means that 148/92 mm Hg meets the criteria for stage 2 hypertension. The other readings provided are within normal limits.

7) C

Explanation: Range of motion exercises should be stopped if the patient voices discomfort and performs gently without force. Active exercises where the patient moves the joint themselves are preferred to passive, and upper and lower extremities can both benefit from range of motion.

91

8) D

Explanation: Patients have a right to receive quality care without discrimination based on race, ethnicity, religion, sex, gender identity, or other personal characteristics. The other options are not guaranteed rights.

9) A

Explanation: The S in SAMPLE stands for symptoms. It reminds the CNA to pay attention to anything the patient is currently experiencing that is out of the ordinary.

10) D

Explanation: Reporting unsafe practices promotes patient safety and reflects ethical behavior. The other options demonstrate unethical actions like avoiding work duties, breaching confidentiality, and working outside of training.

11) A

Explanation: OSHA grants healthcare workers the right to adequate personal protective equipment to minimize workplace hazards and injuries. The other options are not guaranteed under OSHA.

12) D

Explanation: Warm, reddened skin could indicate a pressure ulcer or other skin issue, so the nurse should be notified immediately. The other symptoms should be reported but do not require urgent notification.

13) C

Explanation: Slurred speech can signal a neurological emergency like a stroke, so the nurse should be notified immediately. Do not delay care by trying to assess or provide interventions beyond notification.

14) D

Explanation: Restraints may be used to safely prevent patient falls, with a proper order, appropriate sizing, and close monitoring. The other situations do not demonstrate proper restraint use.

15) B

Explanation: Leaving patient charts or information visible to others who are not involved in care is a breach of confidentiality. The other actions either facilitate care or are allowed with patient permission.

16) D

Explanation: Only RNs and LPNs may accept verbal orders from physicians. The nursing assistant should have the nurse take the verbal order instead.

17) B

Explanation: Regular flexion of the hips and knees helps prevent contractures by maintaining joint mobility and range of motion. This is a key task to perform on bedridden patients.

18) C

Explanation: Patient autonomy relates to the right of patients to make their own healthcare decisions, which is a rights-based ethical concern. The other options do not directly relate to patient rights.

19) A

Explanation: Helping a patient with hygiene before an exam demonstrates caring by providing comfort. Debating treatments, doing unrelated tasks on break, and calling in sick do not reflect caring behaviors.

20) A

Explanation: Key characteristics for patient communication include patience, understanding, and active listening skills to provide compassionate care. Appearance, posture, humor, and speed are less critical.

# EXAM 2 - CORRECT ANSWERS

1) B

Explanation: Measuring and recording urine output provides information about kidney function and hydration status. It does not directly relate to catheter needs or continence training.

2) C

Explanation: Thickened liquids are harder to aspirate. Aspiration involves inhaling food/fluid into the lungs and occurs more readily in patients with impaired gag reflexes. Positioning upright doesn't necessarily prevent it.

3) B

Explanation: LPNs are licensed to perform skilled procedures like wound care. The nursing assistant should offer to assist the LPN if needed. There is no need to remind, report, or document about the appropriate scope.

4) D

Explanation: After verifying a patient is unresponsive, the immediate next action should be to contact emergency medical services by calling for help. Do not attempt to rouse or treat the patient yourself.

5) A

Explanation: Encouraging participation in group activities and social stimulation helps prevent isolation and depression in long-term care patients. The other options will not help prevent depression.

6) B

Explanation: As dementia patients require round-the-clock supervision and long-term care as they can deteriorate, if they live outside of their homes and not with family, they usually live in a nursing home, which can provide those services.

7) C

Explanation: Reporting unsafe conditions promotes patient advocacy and is ethically required. Sharing pictures, working outside of training, and disagreeing with the team are unethical.

8) B

Explanation: Offering the patient dignity by asking if more time or privacy would help meet toileting needs shows compassion. Arguing, threats, or reporting do not diffuse frustration.

9) A

Explanation: For bedrest patients, active motion aimed at joint limits without forcing is ideal. Passive motion provides less benefit, and the upper and lower extremities both need to be exercised.

10) D

Explanation: Chin level position allows patients, particularly those with weakness, to eat with minimal assistance. It does not necessarily exercise arms or teach manners.

11) A

Explanation: Information should only be shared with providers directly involved in the patient's care, following privacy laws. Opinions about others should be avoided.

12) C

Explanation: Limit handoff to factual data about care and status. Opinions about care should be shared directly with the assigned nurse, not passing assistants.

13) B

Explanation: Identifying and quickly reporting safety risks shows responsible advocacy. Only perform delegated tasks, document independently, and contact providers directly if needed.

14) C

Explanation: Empathetic communication conveys compassion. Academic knowledge, reserved manners, and talkative nature are fewer essential traits.

15) C

Explanation: Early pressure ulcers appear as reddened skin that blanches, becoming white with pressure. Pain, edema, and blisters indicate more advanced ulcers.

16) D

Explanation: Assess pulse and call 911 before beginning CPR when finding an unresponsive person. Do not delay this to clear vomit or provide breaths.

17) D

Explanation: Nursing assistants provide mouth care, including brushing, flossing, and denture cleaning. Assessing tissues, obtaining orders, and suctioning exceed the scope of practice.

18) D

Explanation: In an emergency, suctioning a tracheostomy would be performed by a nurse. A nursing assistant can assist by gathering supplies. Absenteeism, deception, and favoritism are unethical.

19) C

Explanation: Concerns about coworker behavior should be shared first with the immediate supervisor before reporting to boards or anonymously. Never solely discuss with peers.

20) B

Explanation: Concerns about other providers' lapses in care should be reported to the manager versus peers, the provider directly, or the medical record.

# EXAM 3 - CORRECT ANSWERS

1) A

Explanation: Acknowledging and documenting errors supports transparency, prevention of recurrence, and integrity. Deception and hiding errors are unethical.

2) A

Explanation: Breaches of confidentiality or privacy must be reported immediately through proper channels, starting with the direct supervisor versus trying to intervene independently.

3) B

Explanation: Unlabeled and unattended medications are unsafe and require immediate disposal. Do not investigate, save, or try to return to staff before disposing properly.

4) C

Explanation: Only document care personally performed. Falsifying or adding to another provider's charting is unethical and illegal.

5) C

Explanation: Concerns should be shared privately up the chain of command, not with the patient. Refusal and sabotage are unethical.

6) A

Explanation: Breaches of privacy/confidentiality must be immediately reported to the direct supervisor. Do not attempt individual interventions like deleting, commenting, or coaching peers.

7) D

Explanation: Documenting errors demonstrates integrity. Lying, hiding errors, or only telling leadership is unethical.

8) B

Explanation: Providing unbiased care, despite personal prejudices, demonstrates beneficence and justice. Reassignment, minimal care, and petitions are unethical.

9) D

Explanation: Nurses' aides may only document the care they personally performed. Signing on another person's behalf is unethical and illegal.

10) A

Explanation: Concerns about privacy breaches require immediate notification of the direct supervisor before other individual interventions.

11) C

Explanation: Suspected abuse must be reported immediately to the appropriate agency. Do not delay, take photos, or try to confirm before reporting.

12) B

Explanation: Questionable practice should be reported immediately before direct intervention with the coworker. Do not delay or confront them directly.

13) C

Explanation: Dysphagia is a swallowing impairment which can lead to choking, aspiration of liquid in the lungs or even bringing food back up. To avoid this, the feeding plan must keep in mind specific food textures.

14) B

Explanation: Performing unauthorized procedures is unsafe and unethical. Reporting safety issues, discussing policies, and properly marking late entries are acceptable.

15) B

Explanation: Suspected impairment concerns should be discreetly reported to leadership versus trying to directly intervene, photograph, or restrict duties independently.

16) B

Explanation: Declining online contacts and sharing personal details maintains appropriate boundaries. After-hours care and promoting independence are appropriate.

17) B

Explanation: After a fall, immediately check for emergency medical alerts, bleeding, and other injuries before moving a person or conducting an interview about what happened.

18) C

Explanation: Caring is shown through compassionate presence without judgment versus fixing, distracting, or reminiscing. Listen fully to expressions of feelings.

19) B

Explanation: Confidentiality must be breached when obligated to report suspected neglect, abuse, or violence to protect the patient's safety.

20) D

Explanation: An ethical response involves honesty, apology, and steps to prevent recurrence. Lying, hiding errors, or only telling leadership is inappropriate.

# EXAM 4 - CORRECT ANSWERS

1) D

Explanation: Checking blood glucose falls within proper nursing assistant training and scope. Catheters, chemotherapy, and central lines require licensed nurse skills.

2) D

Explanation: Reporting unsafe practices reflects principles of justice and beneficence and is ethically required. Social media breaches confidentiality. Care refusal and using internet training are unethical.

3) C

Explanation: In a passive range of motion, the nursing assistant moves the patient's body parts through the joint's range. These maintain flexibility but do not strengthen muscles like active exercises. Slow, gentle motions are used without forcing joints.

4) B

Explanation: After finding a fallen resident, the first priority is assessing for any injuries needing immediate treatment before moving them. Do not attempt to lift or interview before completing this initial assessment.

5) D

Explanation: Nursing assistants can request advance directives indicating residents' wishes. Only nurses/physicians can access power of attorney, DNRs, and guardianships.

6) D

Explanation: Nursing assistants can provide partial feeding assistance to residents. Thickening liquids, assessing swallowing ability, and obtaining diet orders from providers all require licensed nursing assessment and judgment.

7) D

Explanation: Identifying and reporting safety issues demonstrates responsible advocacy for patients. Gossiping, posting private information, or working outside the scope of training would be unethical.

8) B

Explanation: Purulent drainage signifies potential infection and should be immediately reported, not cleaned. Standard or transmission-based precautions are always required for dressings.

9) D

Explanation: Advocating for safety and optimal care demonstrates ethical integrity. Absenteeism, working beyond scope, and care refusal based on bias are unethical.

10) B

Explanation: Fruity breath odor in a diabetic signals ketoacidosis, an emergency. Notify the nurse right away before intervening independently.

11) B

Explanation: After securing a scene, immediately assess a potentially injured or unresponsive person for vital signs and life threats. Do not rush movement or leave before this assessment.

12) A

Explanation: Entering rooms without warning breaches physical privacy. Medical records access, safety measures, and charting are not privacy violations.

13) D

Explanation: Nursing assistants can apply non-sterile warm compresses. Oxygen, sterile dressings, and tube insertions require LPN's scope of practice and training.

14) A

Explanation: Nursing assistants should be prepared for these situations and be ready to be compassionate and patient in their demeanor, never getting offended or upset that they are not remembered. Speaking to them calmly and explaining all the steps is the best approach.

15) B

Explanation: The patient who requires a bedpan has a more urgent need and risks soiling themselves.

16) D

Explanation: Nursing assistants can assist nurses in gathering supplies but cannot change the dressings themselves. Orders must be given directly from a physician to the nurse, so nursing assistants should never relay orders.

17) A

Explanation: When a patient does not move regularly, the muscles can atrophize, which means that they lose strength and volume. They will require assistance in ambulation and maybe other ADLs until physical therapists and/or doctors instruct otherwise.

18) C

Explanation: The Heimlich Maneuver uses thrusts to the higher abdomen inwards and upwards to help dislodge any object or food that is blocking the airway. It is performed by embracing the person from behind and around the waist.

19) A

Explanation: Nursing assistants typically work where short or long-term care is given to people with specific needs. Dentists' offices specifically treat teeth and do not require the services of a nursing assistant.

20) D

Explanation: Documenting errors demonstrates integrity. Lying, hiding errors, or only telling leadership is unethical.

21) D

Explanation: Divulging rumors or confidential information, calling in sick falsely, and preferential are violates ethics. Reporting problems demonstrates ethical practice.

22) B

Explanation: When dressing, always start gently from the stronger side, while when undressing, start from the weaker side, but never rush. If you feel the weather might be too cold or warm, check with the nurse first before changing anything on the patient's care plan.

# Practical Skill Scenarios for Hands-On Preparation

In addition to the written exam, the CNA test includes an evaluation of hands-on caregiving skills. Examiners will direct candidates to perform 5-6 procedural tasks representing knowledge of real-world techniques, safety, and competence. This section provides examples of the practical skill scenarios tested to help build hands-on abilities.

Some of the skills present will require direct performance, while others will be verbal descriptions of the procedures. Examiners will provide equipment and materials as needed for the demonstrated tasks.

## *Sample Skills Scenario #1*

Handwashing

- The examiner will ask you to demonstrate proper handwashing techniques. Explain each step of the process as you demonstrate washing hands correctly. You will be observed for proper technique and use of supplies.

Mouth Care

- The examiner will provide a toothbrush, a small cup of water, a sink, and a privacy curtain. Demonstrate how you will provide mouth care for a resident who cannot get out of bed, including gathering supplies, providing for privacy, cleaning teeth properly, maintaining safety throughout, and leaving the resident comfortable. Explain your actions to the examiner.

Feeding a Dependent Resident

- Demonstrate how you would assist a resident who cannot feed themselves to eat their meal. The examiner will act as the resident. Explain your actions, including preparation, safety, ensuring adequate intake, and maintaining dignity.

## *Sample Skills Scenario #2*

Ambulating a Resident with a Cane

- Demonstrate how to ambulate a resident who uses a cane for stability. The examiner will act as the resident. Explain your actions, including preparing the resident, the proper way to hold and use a cane, assisting techniques, safety, and providing for rest periods.

Perineal Care for Incontinent Resident

- Explain steps you would take to provide perineal care for an incontinent resident who is unable to carry out their own toileting hygiene. Clarify preparation, safety, infection prevention, use of materials, proper cleansing motions, and restoring resident's comfort when finished.

Range of Motion Exercise

- Select a joint and demonstrate how to take a resident through a range of motion exercises for that joint. Explain your actions, including safety, gentle movements, technique to support the joint, and signs of pain or discomfort to stop exercise.

## Sample Skills Scenario #3

Weighing an Ambulatory Resident

- Demonstrate how you will properly weigh a resident who can walk but needs some assistance. Explain your actions, including safety, preparing scale, assisting residents, accurate recording, and ensuring resident stability throughout. The examiner will act as the resident.

Measuring and Recording Respirations

- Demonstrate how to properly measure and record a resident's respirations. Explain your actions, including preparation, placing your hand on the resident's chest, counting method, length of time, and recording. The examiner will act as the resident.

Donning and Removing PPE

- Explain the full sequence of steps you would follow to correctly put on, wear, and remove personal protective equipment. The examiner will provide a gown, gloves, surgical mask, and face shield for you to demonstrate proper donning and doffing.

# Conclusion

We have now come full circle on an incredible journey of growth. From foundational concepts to advanced skills, you have traversed the comprehensive arc of knowledge needed for CNA certification exam mastery. More importantly, you have cultivated the understanding required to thrive in this meaningful role centered on caring for others.

Whether fresh out of high school or navigating a mid-life career change, you chose this guide as a stepping stone to success. Now, you stand fully prepared, with the tools needed to pass the exam and flourish in your service. You have built clinical expertise through step-by-step technique instructions. Legal and ethical matters help guide your actions. Communication and behavioral strategies empower you to see the person behind each patient.

Ultimately, though, no exam can test the empathy in your heart that sparked this pursuit to begin with. That human quality of compassion is what truly fuels excellence in this work. You are now equipped to channel that care into masterfully executed interventions that improve quality of life. That personal drive to help others is your most precious asset.

Of course, as in any profession, true expertise only comes through practice and experience. Passing the certification exam is just the first milestone on an exciting road of continual growth. Formally entering the healthcare field is when the theories transform into practical realities. Be receptive to learning as much from seasoned CNA partners as from your initial training. Bring an open mind and know there are always new lessons to absorb. Remember, too, that caregiving can be as rewarding for the giver as for the recipient, but it can also be emotionally draining at times. Draw healthy boundaries and practice self-care to avoid burnout. Your well-being directly impacts patients – you cannot pour from an empty vessel. Seek support from both supervisors and peers. And take pride in the privilege of being entrusted with other people's most vulnerable moments.

As you embark on your new career, hold close to the core those principles that brought you here: to provide care rooted in compassion, communication, ethics, safety, and skill. Build on that foundation each day through practical experience. Aspire to ever greater competence while retaining the empathy that grounds your work. The two must go hand-in-hand for care to be transformative.

You now stand ready to begin an incredible journey. One where small everyday acts of caring can change lives, improve well-being, and affirm humanity for both the giver and receiver. Not only will you pass the exam, but you will excel at uplifting others. You will help countless individuals navigate seasons of vulnerability with dignity, optimism, and grace.

This is the opportunity of a lifetime – to be a light for others in distressing times of illness or frailty. To escort them along difficult but meaningful passages of life. What an honor to be entrusted with people's most fragile moments. And what a chance to reap the rewards that come from serving with an open heart.

Go forward then, in hope. The knowledge you need is now within grasp. When exam day arrives, be confident in all you have prepared for. Stay calm and focused, and trust your abilities. Visualize walking out certified, qualified, and exhilarated to begin this work you felt drawn towards. Now, go out and bless the world with exactly the care it needs. Your contributions will be invaluable.

# EXTRA CONTENT DOWNLOAD

This is my way of saying thank you
to my loyal readers!
SCAN THE QR-CODE BELOW
TO DOWNLOAD YOUR EXTRA CONTENT!

Should you encounter any issues downloading it, please write to:

nathanyarbridge@gmail.com – our team will send it to you.

As in any growth journey, your feedback is invaluable.

I invite you to share your opinion by leaving a review of this book on Amazon.com

SCAN THE QRCODE

THANK YOU FOR YOUR SUPPORT, IT'S TRULY VALUABLE TO ME!

Follow the social page of our international community

by clicking on the QR codes below, for updates, news, and surprises!

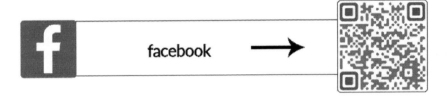

Made in the USA
Middletown, DE
19 June 2025

77235164R00062